Emphysema

and

Chronic Obstructive Pulmonary Disease

Therapeutic Approaches Through

Nutrition

Natural Medicine

Alternative Medicine

Robert J. Green Jr., N.D.

Aventine Press

Aventine Press
1023 4th Avenue
204
San Diego, CA 92101

Library of Congress Control Number: 2005935714

Library of Congress Cataloging-in-Publication Data:

Green, Jr., Robert J., 1962-
        Emphysema and Chronic Obstructive Pulmonary Disease
        Therapeutic Approaches Through: Nutrition, Natural Medicine,
        Alternative Medicine

ISBN: 1-59330-332-7

1. Emphysema and COPD – Popular works. 2. Emphysema and COPD – Nutritional therapeutics. 3. Emphysema and COPD – Natural medicine. 4. Emphysema and COPD – Alternative medicine.

Manuscript edited by Stephen Llevares.

Illustrations and cover art provided by Dan Woodward.

The author may be contacted through the publisher, or via e-mail at:
emphysemabookcomments@yahoo.com

Visit the World Wide Web at:
www.emphysemabook.net

Printed in the United States of America

To my father, Robert Green Sr., whose personal battle with laryngeal cancer and COPD inspired the writing of this book.

To my wife, Patricia, whose virtue no words can describe, and my children, John, Zarah, and Joseph, you are my joy.

To Mr. and Mrs. Francesco Caccavale, without whose support the final writing of this manuscript could have never occurred.

And to the Lord, in whom all healing is found. You are my light and my truth.

Table of Contents

Figures and Tables

Note to the Reader

The purpose of this book is to serve as an accurate and authoritative reference with regard to the subject material presented. The information presented in this book is a scholarly treatise that has been compiled from the author's academic study and personal experience. The author is not a physician. The material presented in this book is for informational and educational purposes only, and not for the rendering of a diagnosis, treatment plan, or medical advice. All measures that you pursue toward improving your health, specifically to include the application or utilization of any material derived from this book, should always first be discussed with your physician and commenced only under the supervision of your physician or other qualified healthcare provider. The information in this text should never be viewed as a substitute for competent care by a qualified healthcare provider. Any statements made by the author with respect to particular products and/or services represent the views of the author alone. The author receives no compensation for the endorsement of any products or services mentioned in this book. The author and the publisher assume no liability, arising either directly or indirectly, from the application or use of any information in this book.

Acknowledgments

My sincerest thanks are given to all my former professors, and also to every person who was instrumental in bringing this manuscript to fruition. The following individuals, however, are deserving of special mention, as their contributions to my life have been invaluable. Collectively they taught me how to think critically, and how to appropriately apply reason in formulating meaningful questions of value. As teachers, their tireless dedication and stellar reputations for academic excellence will forever remain the bar against which I measure myself. But perhaps more importantly, through the impact of their kindness and selfless humility, I became a better person by knowing them. For all they have given me, I am forever grateful.

Robert F. Good, M.D.
(In Memoriam)

Herbert Lebherz, Ph.D.
Professor Emeritus of Biochemistry

John Kotselas, M.A.
Author and Lecturer in Theology

William Cheek, Ph.D.
Professor Emeritus of History

Sharon Satterfield, N.D.
Doctor of Naturopathy

Henry Shatz, M.A.
Professor of Spanish

Hans Behrisch, Ph.D.
Professor of Biochemistry

About the Author

Robert Green Jr. is a traditional naturopath, health researcher, and an author. He received the Associate of Arts (A.A.) degree in liberal arts from San Diego City College in 1995, and the Bachelor of Arts (B.A.) degree from San Diego State University in 1998. At San Diego State University he majored in religious studies and minored in human biology and pre–medicine, and throughout his academic life he has continuously studied the areas of mathematics, physics, chemistry and biochemistry, cellular and molecular biology, and the health sciences.

In 1994 he began to study nutrition along with natural and alternative therapeutics in an effort to help his father who had been diagnosed with laryngeal cancer and chronic obstructive pulmonary disease. Following graduation from college, he attended medical school; however, a mounting interest in the application of nutritional and natural health principles to chronic obstructive pulmonary disease, along with evolving family responsibilities, led to the decision to complete the doctor of naturopathy (N.D.) degree through Trinity College of Natural Health.

Trinity College of Natural Health, located in Warsaw, Indiana, is accredited by the American Naturopathic Medical Accreditation Board, and is one of America's leading nontraditional colleges of nutrition and natural health that seeks to preserve the knowledge of natural health principles and techniques that have served humanity throughout the world. Dr. Green also holds professional memberships with the American Association of Drugless Practitioners and the American Alternative Medical Association.

In keeping with his commitment to the highest ideals of scholarship, and to further understand the molecular and biophysical bases of health and disease, Dr. Green continues to study current research findings from the two main areas of investigation within the biological/health sciences and natural/alternative therapeutics: basic science research that is aimed at elucidating underlying molecular, cellular, and systemic mechanisms, as well as clinical research efforts that are demonstrating the greatest promise toward being efficacious in bringing about positive changes in human health.

So as to ensure a comprehensive perspective, a multidisciplinary approach is applied — one that combines information from a variety of disciplines so as to produce an integrated framework of knowledge that functions together in the quest to find answers to the important questions regarding the biological and energetic processes that are essential to human life. Such an integrated approach enables the development of a broader understanding of the fundamental mechanisms of action of molecules and energy in living systems as well as the interplay between the molecules and energy that are involved in the myriad of issues in human health today.

Preface

A major paradigm shift is occurring across the healthcare landscape today. The development of the Internet over the last two decades has provided unprecedented accessibility to information like never before in history. This broad access to information has contributed greatly to increasing people's knowledge in a myriad of areas, but in the area of health in particular, the tremendous amount of information disseminated through the Internet has left people today with many choices to meet their healthcare needs that only a generation ago were nonexistent.

In this present day and age of health freedom and increased awareness of healthcare, people are realizing that the options available to them to build health and prevent illness reach far beyond the borders of conventional medicine. People today know that prescription drugs and surgery, although well warranted in some instances, are often not the solution to their problems. Today's informed consumer knows that nutrition can play a significant role in addressing their health concerns, and this is especially important when dealing with emphysema and COPD (chronic obstructive pulmonary disease). Knowledge of the therapeutic use of nutritional supplements and herbs, for example, that until a decade or so ago was only known in esoteric circles, is now making its way well into the mainstream. People are becoming more and more aware of the use of homeopathy to build health, and current research reminds us to never underestimate the merits of proper exercise. The therapeutic value of acupuncture has become so well recognized that it is essentially as much a part of the mainstream as chiropractic. In general, the flood of information that has occurred through the Internet and the media has enabled people to know that there is a whole world of knowledge out there that can be put to use to help with the issues of their health.

The conventional healthcare system is beginning to embrace a principle that has always been part of natural health practice, and that is the idea that healthcare involves building the health and wellness of the whole person, not just treating their immediate symptoms. The methods of natural health are tailored and applied to meet an individual's overall needs, and in so doing not only are their immediate concerns addressed, but the entirety of their well-being is considered so as to enable them to have a steady, positive progression toward greater health to the maximum extent that they are capable.

With the vast amount of information that is available today on health and healing, people often become bewildered with the enormity of choices they have. Making sense of all this information is often the reason why an individual turns to a natural health practitioner for help. As individuals increasingly continue to trust in natural health practitioners to guide and educate them through their choices, it is incumbent upon those practitioners to exercise the highest levels of integrity, academic scrutiny, and sound, educated judgment when consulting with these individuals. It is with those precepts in mind that this book is offered.

Depending upon the extent of your academic background, some of the material may present challenges in reading. I have simplified the presentation of the material as much as possible; however, anatomy, physiology and pathology are what they are, and in my commitment to make this book comprehensive and thorough, it was necessary to include this material. Another commitment I made in writing this book was to not only present the protocols that have the highest potential for success in addressing COPD through nutritional and natural therapeutics, but to always provide an adequate explanation of why these protocols are believed to be useful. I believe that every individual has a right to not only fully understand their condition as best as they are able, but that they should also be provided with an understanding of the rationale behind any treatment protocols they are either using or considering. Some of the explanations of nutritional protocols and the use of supplements and herbs are somewhat detailed. In order to assist you with any potentially unfamiliar scientific or medically related vocabulary, I have defined many terms as they appear in the text. I have also included a glossary at the end of the book.

Enjoy the journey through this book. There is a lot of information here that can make a positive difference in your health and your life. May you be blessed and encouraged as you begin the process to build your health.

Introduction

It is estimated that approximately 35 million people in the United States have been diagnosed with one of the forms of COPD. As the fourth leading cause of death in America, COPD claims nearly 120,000 lives annually. The number of people diagnosed with COPD worldwide is as high as 293 million. Despite the best of intentions, conventional medicine is still limited in what it can offer to help with the problem of COPD, and when we consider the magnitude of the abovementioned statistics, there inherently exists an overwhelming need to look at the issue of emphysema/COPD from an alternative and natural health perspective. The need for an alternative view is all the more compelling when we also consider that as a nation we spent more than 37 billion dollars on COPD care in 2004. I subscribe to the idea that the knowledge and methods of nutrition and natural health should be made not only accessible but also sought after by both the general public and the professional healthcare community. Therefore by means of this logical, evaluative, and unbiased text, I undertook to present in an honest and well-substantiated manner the current understanding of the therapeutic approaches to COPD through nutrition and natural/alternative therapeutics. It is my hope that this treatise will be welcomed in an effort to help improve the lives of the countless millions of individuals suffering from the depredation of this condition. Only through developing an integrative model of care that is served by health educators and practitioners with open minds and cooperative dispositions who avoid the trappings of political and intellectual quagmires will the comprehensive health needs of human beings ultimately be met.

Living with the ravages of COPD is no way to live, and dying from COPD is on the highest order of menacing. This condition doesn't just take you — it takes its time with you and puts you through hell and back as it slowly, and with much misery and discomfort, suffocates you. A graphic portrayal perhaps, but an honest one nonetheless, as there is no reason to be other than direct when dealing with something this serious. For those of us who have either lived with, or personally taken care of someone with COPD, we know all too well the very high price these individuals pay in their daily attempts to just survive and have a halfway decent quality of life.

My interest and subsequent passion to help people with this condition began a little over a decade ago as I started to watch the effects of COPD take hold of my own father. As I took care of him and became more and more involved with researching alternatives to help, the career path in conventional medicine that I had envisioned as a youth took on a new face as I began to discover the vast realm of knowledge on healing and science that was beyond the domain of what would be considered mainstream orthodox medical thinking. Although my years of study and research drew upon both conventional and natural/alternative paradigms, I came to have a great appreciation for the natural health paradigm as it not only demonstrated to have a considerable variety of means by which to offer help, it also showed that it could be very efficacious in bringing about improvement; it always addressed people's health within the larger context of their whole person — not just their immediate complaints or issues. I sincerely value the merits of modern medicine and humbly submit that conventional medicine plays a very noteworthy role in helping those with emphysema/COPD; however, it was the integration of nutritional and natural therapeutics that made the most significant difference in my father's life. At 82 my father is still with us, and although he is toward the end of his plight with COPD, it was the integration of natural therapeutics that has given him a veritable quality of life for these last 10 years.

Reflecting on the research and study I have done throughout these years has enabled me to recognize that I am truly a scientist and researcher at heart. I have come to thoroughly enjoy the puzzle solving and scientific detective work inherent in research for it not only provides us with increased knowledge and understanding into the inner workings of nature, but moreover that knowledge very often has practical implications that enables clinicians to better serve and help improve the lives of individuals. If I may parenthetically insert here to anyone reading this who is contemplating a career in biological or nutritional science; the opportunities are numerous for those who are interested in researching the fundamental role of nutrition in biological systems as well as determining the mechanisms of action of nutritional and natural therapeutics as they relate to human health and disease. Working in this growing and rewarding field will enable you to solve problems and find solutions to many of the issues in health-related research today, and in so doing you will contribute to making a positive impact on the health of countless numbers of lives.

This book is written primarily for individuals that have already been diagnosed by a physician with chronic obstructive pulmonary disease who are interested in learning about the information that is available regarding nutritional healing and natural/alternative therapeutics, and who desire to employ natural health principles to build up their health. While I have endeavored to keep scholarly language to a minimum, there is still sufficient detail such that this text will be quite useful to professors and students, and practical to practicing naturopaths as well as medical doctors and osteopathic physicians with a penchant for natural health principles as they face the challenges of treating COPD in their practices. This book is by no means intended to represent itself as an exhaustive source of all that could be known about the respiratory system or COPD. Nor is it meant to insinuate that natural or alternative therapeutics is a panacea for this otherwise complex and sophisticated condition that is presently not considered curable. Rather, it seeks to give an overview of that which is currently understood regarding COPD, followed by an in-depth exploration of the means, methods, and philosophies specific to nutrition and natural/alternative therapeutics that have shown themselves to be efficacious in helping to improve the lives of individuals who are living with the consequences of emphysema/COPD.

This first edition of *Emphysema and Chronic Obstructive Pulmonary Disease — Therapeutic Approaches Through: Nutrition, Natural Medicine, Alternative Medicine* fills a great void in the literature as it is the first full-length text devoted solely to COPD that discusses the subject extensively from the viewpoint of nutrition and natural/alternative therapeutics. The research and sources upon which the information in this book is based are both vast and diverse. An impeccable bibliography is included to support and substantiate the information given; every attempt has been made to exclude anecdotal evidence and to only present information that has either been substantiated by valid scientific research or that has historically stood the test of time.

Natural health as a concept has been around for as long as human civilization has existed. As a defined category of health practice, it has a history that slightly exceeds 100 years. The increased interest within many of today's scientific and academic circles over the role that nutrition and natural therapeutics play in human health has prompted an increase in availability of grant funding for the study of nutrition and natural substances in our universities and research institutes. Many of the outcomes of these studies that are occurring with herbs, for example, are confirming that which has been known empirically throughout history. Current research efforts today are also bringing about the discovery of new applications of herbs and supplements as well as fundamental information on the roles that nutrients play in human metabolism.

Always at the heart of the natural health paradigm, though, is a focus on building health, and not just the management or treatment of disease. Proponents of natural health practices have always understood that when you focus on building health by eliminating toxicities and giving the body what it needs to properly function, the problems that conventional medicine refers to as disease oftentimes resolve themselves. America has spoken in regard to her attitude toward natural and alternative healthcare. At the end of 2002, Americans were making more visits to alternative and natural health practitioners than they were to conventional doctors. They spent around 30 billion dollars out-of-pocket for approximately 600 million office visits. In response to the millions of individuals and their families who suffer with COPD who count themselves among those who are sincerely seeking answers and help from the arena of natural and alternative therapeutics, this book is offered to you with the hope that it will help ease your suffering and enable you to learn how to build real health to the extent that you are able — such that you may attain to a quality of life that you otherwise may have never envisioned, given the predicament you face.

We all have choices to make everyday. If you are like the vast majority of people who have been diagnosed with COPD, it is because at some point in your life you made the choice to smoke. Appendix 2 at the end of this book will address the issue of smoking cessation, but it is well worth saying here in the introduction that if you are diagnosed with emphysema/COPD and you are still smoking, then you absolutely must make an earnest effort to stop, because at this point all the help in the world will be of little good to you if you don't stop smoking. I watched cigarettes kill my mother, I'm still witnessing what they did to my father, and believe it or not, I used to smoke myself. I know how hard it is to quit, and I will discuss this in the appendix, but please understand that without quitting cigarettes, your healing process will never begin. Taking steroids and bronchodilators and oxygen does not constitute healing. Yes, they are awfully important in their own right in that they perform an important job for you that is oftentimes critical in sustaining your life, but that is all they are meant to do. And, as important as they are, in the bigger scheme of things these drugs will never move you in the direction of improved health and vitality. They will simply aid you in maintaining your status quo. Changing your attitude and your behavior is the true beginning of healing. The battleground of healing is in your mind. For that matter, even though there is a strong physical addiction component to smoking, the majority of the cigarette battle is in your mind. You already know this. You must acquire control over your mind and your will in order to stop smoking. I'll say it again: You have to stop smoking if you haven't already done so.

As for the battle to rebuild your health beginning in your mind, think back to the day you were sitting in your physician's office and were given the news of being diagnosed with COPD. Unless you are part of the 10–15 percent of COPD cases that are not smoking related, you may have begun to blame yourself for something that you could have otherwise prevented. You've now come to realize there is only so much your physician can do to help you with the consequences of this problem. He or she has been prescribing drugs to help you with your symptoms, but ultimately you have to recognize that how you emerge from this is entirely up to you. You have no time to waste blaming yourself or wishing you could go back and do things differently. What's done is done. You cannot allow yourself to become hindered by negative thoughts that will enter into your mind and try to rob you of essential energy that you now need in order to keep yourself focused on the pathway of rebuilding your health and your life. You are in a fight now, and — make no mistake about it – a fight with emphysema/COPD is absolutely no matter to take lightly. Whether or not you consciously choose to pursue a life of health and wellness will entirely determine how the rest of your life progresses.

Once you change your mind and begin purposing yourself to cultivate a life of wellness and vitality rather than just coping with the consequences of this disease, you can then begin taking the practical steps aimed at building your health. One of the greatest things you can do for yourself is to learn as much as you can about this condition and then arm yourself with as much information as possible on healing. Within this book I will not only share with you what I know, but I will point you to where you can find out more. The realm of natural and alternative healing is vast, and I encourage you to explore all legitimate avenues that offer hope in helping you with your condition.

With proper guidance from your healthcare provider, you can begin to incorporate the things you are about to learn from this book into your life. You will learn about eating correctly as it relates to your health in general and in particular to your COPD, as well as how to use specific foods therapeutically. As you become more involved and focused on your health and building wellness, you'll start to appreciate how herbs and nutritional supplements can be applied to improve your momentum toward greater health and well-being. You will discover how the techniques of acupuncture and chiropractic care can enhance your condition, and you will hopefully acquire an understanding of how valuable a skilled homeopathic practitioner can be in helping you to restore your health to its maximum potential. If you are faithful to consistently apply natural health principles to your life, you'll begin to see improvements in other areas of your life and health such that you'll come to realize that what I am writing about goes beyond just trying to ease the complications that are associated with your emphysema/COPD.

Always bear in mind that natural health as a concept is a way of life, not just a way of healing illness. It is a set of principles that invokes our need to recognize the necessity of living a balanced life as the best means to promote a healthy existence. The modern American lifestyle is often at odds with these principles, but with the rampage of chronic disease and other health conditions in this country that were essentially unheard of years ago, one can only logically surmise that the time is long overdue for us to adopt a healthier way of living. We can no longer continue to live in a manner that overlooks our personal responsibility towards our health by thinking that it is modern medicine's job to rescue us from everything that befalls us. Modern medicine serves us in many important ways, but never to the exclusion of our personal responsibility for our health. I trust you will eventually emerge with a heightened awareness of the accountability we all have towards our health, a renewed respect for the privilege of having been given this life in the first place, and lastly a genuine appreciation for the trust that has been placed in all of us to properly steward this life we have been given.

†Robert Green Jr.
Long Island, N.Y.
July 2005

Chapter 1

Essential Respiratory Anatomy and Physiology

Introduction

Overall, the main purpose of the lungs is to facilitate the exchange of carbon dioxide for oxygen. In so doing the lungs fulfill a crucial role in the first two phases of respiration, a four-phase process whereby life-sustaining oxygen is delivered to the cells of the body while the cellular metabolic waste product carbon dioxide is simultaneously removed. The first phase of respiration is breathing, otherwise known as pulmonary ventilation, or the inspiration (inhaling) and expiration (exhaling) of air. Breathing is controlled by the medulla oblongata and the pons, structures located in the brain stem portion of the central nervous system, through nerve impulses that stimulate the appropriate thoracic muscles and the diaphragm. The second phase is external (pulmonary) respiration, where the exchange of gases (oxygen and carbon dioxide) occurs between the lungs and the blood. Oxygen transfer from the lungs into the blood in the second phase of respiration is always dependent upon there being sufficient amounts of hemoglobin in the blood; in cases where hemoglobin is lower than optimal (as with anemia), there can be additional concerns for persons with COPD. The third phase of respiration, which does not occur in the lungs, is called internal (tissue) respiration, and it involves the exchange of gases between the blood and the tissues. The final phase of respiration, cellular respiration, occurs inside the cells of the body. Through the process of cellular respiration, the oxygen that has been obtained from the blood is used by the cells of the body to make energy and sustain metabolic activity, and in the course of so doing, carbon dioxide is generated as a waste product.

The life and well-being of the entire body are vitally dependent upon proper and efficient functioning of every detail of respiration. The respiratory system must not only operate efficiently, but it must also protect itself from environmental irritants and infection. Emphysema and COPD present various and sizeable problems involving the first two phases of respiration, and moreover, the problems of emphysema and COPD can be further complicated when there are also concurrent problems with the heart, liver, kidneys, or intestines. This book will endeavor to discuss the wide range of problems associated with COPD and will elaborate at length on what help can be offered through nutrition and natural/alternative therapeutics. In order to make the material on therapeutics more meaningful, a brief elemental overview of anatomy and physiology will now be presented so as to provide a basic working knowledge of the structure and function of the respiratory system.

General anatomy of the lungs

The lungs themselves are very elastic sponge-like organs that lie in the thoracic cavity. The lungs are enclosed within the ribcage with the apex of the lungs (most superior part) reaching just slightly above the clavicle (collar bone), and the base of the lungs, which is slightly curved, fits over the curved area of the diaphragm. The right lung is somewhat shorter than the left so as to accommodate the space needed by the liver that lies just below the diaphragm under the right lung. A two-layered serous membrane composed mainly of elastic tissue known as the pleural membrane encloses and protects the lungs within the thoracic cavity. The inner membrane, the visceral pleura, lines the lungs themselves, whereas the outer layer, the parietal pleura, is attached to the thoracic wall. A thin film of serous fluid (pleural fluid in this case) occupies the space between the two membranes in order that the two membranous surfaces (the visceral and parietal pleura) can easily slide over one another during inspiration and expiration. The right lung consists of three lobes and the left lung has two. Additionally, the right lung is divided into ten sections and the left lung into nine. These sections amount to what can be thought of as a three-dimensional map that enables greater precision in defining anatomical location. This is very practical when attempting to determine the locus of a problem in the lungs. Figure 1 illustrates the overall respiratory system and related structures, and will serve as a useful general reference.

Figure 1 **Illustration of the respiratory system and related structures.**

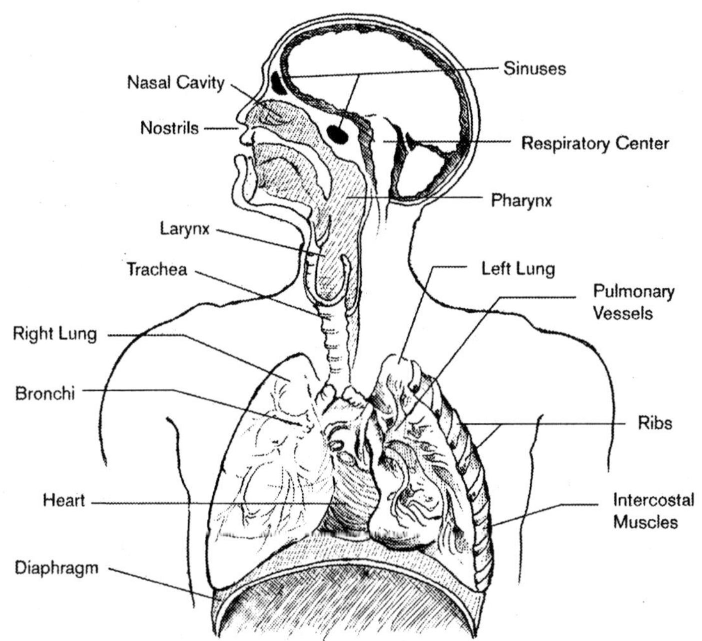

Pathway of airflow through the respiratory system

The respiratory system begins at the anterior nares (nostrils), where air enters the nasal cavity and proceeds by way of the nasal meatuses through the posterior nares (choanae) into the nasopharynx. As air passes through the structures of the nasal cavity, it is filtered by coarse nasal hairs, and warmed and humidified by a highly vascularized mucous membrane. More will be said later regarding the role of the mucous membranes found throughout the respiratory tract. From the nasopharynx, air continues onward down the oropharynx and the laryngopharynx (essentially the back of the mouth and the throat) through the larynx (voice box) into the trachea. The trachea (windpipe) is a cartilaginous tube that extends down from the larynx about 4½ inches where it then bifurcates (divides into two branches) into the right and left primary bronchi (first two main branches of the bronchial tree). Now at the threshold of entering the lungs proper, the air that initially began at the anterior nares will soon find its way into the alveoli (air sacs) of the lungs by way of an elaborate system of branches that are collectively known as bronchi and bronchioles.

When the primary bronchi enter the lungs, they begin branching to form smaller bronchi called secondary or lobar bronchi. The secondary (lobar) bronchi continue to divide and branch to become tertiary bronchi, which further divide to become bronchioles. Bronchioles eventually become terminal bronchioles (less than 2mm in diameter) that give rise to branches of respiratory bronchioles (alveoli appear at this level), which divide into alveolar ducts and ultimately end as clusters of alveolar sacs with their respective alveoli. Alveolar sacs are simply two or more alveoli that share a common opening from an alveolar duct. Terminal bronchioles along with their respective respiratory bronchioles and their distal alveolar sacs and alveoli are known as lobules. Respiratory bronchioles along with their distal alveolar sacs and alveoli are collectively known as the acinus. The acinus is essentially a lobule without including the terminal bronchiole, and the acinus is the pulmonary functional unit where actual gas exchange occurs. Metaphorically speaking, the acinus can be likened to a cluster of grapes where the main stem coming off the vine is the respiratory bronchiole, the smaller stems are the alveolar ducts, and the grapes themselves represent the alveoli. This comparison of the acinus to a cluster of grapes is of course by no means perfectly analogous to the actual structure of the acinus, but it is nonetheless a worthwhile example to illustrate the idea of the overall schema of what the acinus looks like.

Table 1 should help give clarity to the pathway of airflow through the respiratory system. Note that numbers 9 through 13 comprise what is referred to as a lobule. Numbers 10 through 13 comprise the acinus. Figure 2 on the next page is an illustration of an electron micrograph showing the architecture of the acinus.

Table 1

Pathway of Airflow Through the Respiratory System

1. Nasal Cavity
2. Pharynx (nasopharynx, oropharynx, laryngopharynx)
3. Larynx
4. Trachea
5. Left and Right Primary Bronchi
6. Secondary (Lobar) Bronchi
7. Tertiary Bronchi
8. Bronchioles

9. Terminal Bronchioles
10. Respiratory Bronchioles
11. Alveolar Ducts
12. Alveolar Sacs
13. Individual Alveoli

9 – 13 = Lobule
10 – 13 = Acinus
(The acinus is the actual site of gas exchange.)

Figure 2 **Illustration of an electron micrograph of a cast of two acini showing a terminal bronchiole splitting into two respiratory bronchioles with their respective alveolar ducts and alveoli.**

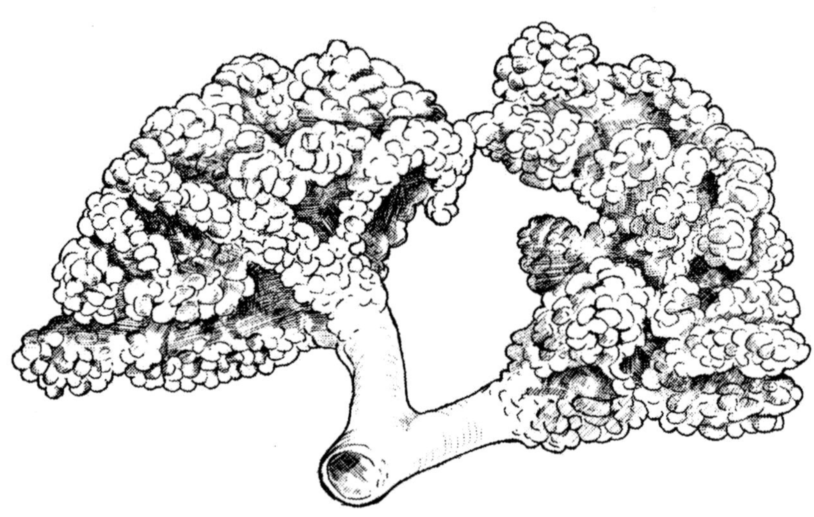

Structural support of the respiratory system

Structural support of the respiratory tract from the trachea to the bronchioles is provided primarily by cartilaginous rings and plates. The cartilaginous rings that provide support in the trachea and primary bronchi are eventually replaced by plates of cartilage as the branching network progresses deeper into the lungs. The cartilage plates disappear in the bronchioles as bronchioles themselves are not supported by cartilage, but rather are surrounded by smooth muscle, which allows for fluctuation in the size of the bronchiole. Bronchioles are also characterized by the presence of elastic fibers that surround the bronchiole in addition to the smooth muscle.

Blood supply to the lungs

There are two separate systems of blood flow in the lungs. The first of these two systems involves the blood that circulates from the heart through the pulmonary vessels. This is the system that is responsible for picking up oxygen from the alveoli so that it can be transported to the tissues throughout the body. As blood circulates throughout the body, the tissues utilize oxygen from the blood for their metabolic needs, and in so doing, the blood that is returned to the heart is essentially without oxygen. This deoxygenated blood is then sent from the heart to the lungs by way of the pulmonary artery where it reaches the capillaries that surround the alveoli. It is at the alveoli/capillary interface that the blood receives a fresh supply of oxygen. After passing through the alveolar capillaries, the freshly oxygenated blood makes its way back to the heart by way of the pulmonary vein where it then exits the heart through the aorta and circulates through another cycle of delivering oxygen to the tissues of the body.

You may have learned that arteries are blood vessels that carry oxygen-rich blood away from the heart and veins are blood vessels that carry oxygen-poor blood from the tissues back to the heart. This is mostly correct. However, be mindful that the definition of an artery or vein hinges on the direction of blood flow (toward or away from the heart), and not on the oxygen content of the blood contained within. The pulmonary artery and vein are exceptions to the norm in that even though the blood in the pulmonary artery is deoxygenated, it is an artery nonetheless as it is carrying blood away from the heart. The pulmonary vein, even though it is carrying oxygen-rich blood as a result of having just picked up oxygen in the alveolar capillaries, is still called a vein because it is taking blood towards the heart.

The second system of blood flow in the lungs is the circulation of blood through the bronchial vessels that nourish the lung tissue itself. The bronchial arteries receive oxygenated blood mainly from the aorta, and deliver this oxygen-rich blood to the lung tissue (e.g. bronchi and bronchioles, visceral pleura, bronchial lymph nodes) via the capillaries that are adjacent to the cells of these tissues. Upon the lung tissue utilizing the oxygen from the bronchial arteries, some of the now deoxygenated blood is returned to the heart by way of the pulmonary veins, as there exists some communication between these two systems of circulation (pulmonary and bronchial), and some of the deoxygenated blood is returned to the heart through the bronchial veins, which are branches of the azygos system.

Lining of the respiratory tract and the alveoli

The nasal cavity and nasopharynx, along with the remainder of the respiratory system from the larynx (not including the vocal chords) to the bronchioles, are lined by a mucous membrane containing what are known as pseudostratified ciliated columnar epithelial cells with many mucous-secreting goblet cells. There are also many submucosal mucous-secreting glands throughout the walls of the trachea and the bronchi, but not the bronchioles. These cells and glands, through the combined mechanical actions of mucus and cilia, accomplish the task of conditioning inspired air and keeping the respiratory system clean and free of particulate matter. Moist mucus secreted by the goblet cells and/or mucous-secreting glands traps foreign matter, while cilia on the epithelium sweeps it away such that it is either swallowed or expectorated. This is the natural course of action for maintaining the respiratory passageways. Water for the humidification of inspired air is derived from mucus, and heat to warm the air is obtained through the abundant underlying blood vessels. These processes work together to ensure that the air that travels through the respiratory tract is not only at body temperature, but also as clean as possible, and completely humidified.

From the bronchioles onward, the branching network becomes very extensive, and the cells lining the respiratory tract gradually begin to change. Upon reaching the terminal bronchioles, the lining of the respiratory tract has changed from pseudostratified ciliated columnar epithelial cells with goblet cells to nonciliated simple cuboidal epithelial cells. At this point the cells lining the respiratory tract no longer produce mucus, nor do they have cilia, and an immune system cell known as a macrophage assumes the responsibility of removing inhaled foreign particles. Rather than trapping and sweeping away foreign matter like cilia, macrophages engulf and digest the foreign particulate matter. As the terminal bronchioles eventually become respiratory bronchioles, the cells lining the respiratory tract change yet again into a cell type known as squamous epithelium, which is consistent with the general structure of the alveolar wall. The alveolar wall itself is composed of a continuous lining of what are known as type 1 alveolar cells (squamous pulmonary epithelial cells) with occasional type 2 alveolar cells (septal cells). Figure 3 will help clarify the cellular changes that occur along the pathway of the respiratory tract.

Figure 3 **Illustration of the general overall changes in the structure of the lining of the respiratory tract.**

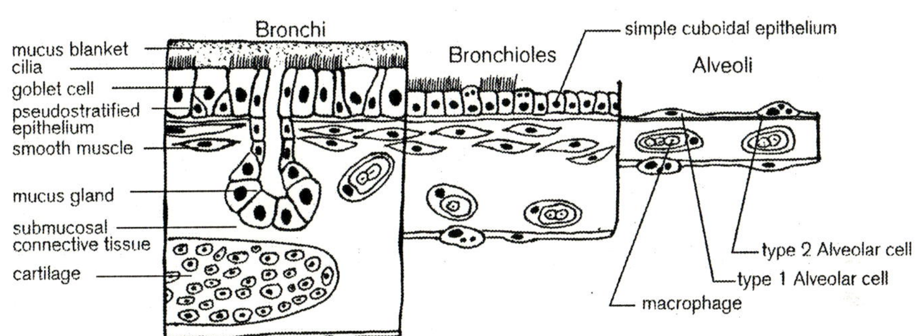

The walls of the alveoli are composed of only a single layer of cells, and they lie immediately adjacent to capillaries that also consist of only a single layer of cells. Each lung has roughly 300 million alveoli and each one of them is essentially a gas bubble that is surrounded by a network of capillaries. The alveolar wall also contains its own macrophages that are responsible for removing dust particles and other debris from the alveoli. With the inner surface of the alveoli being moist as well as having direct contact with air (gas), the watery surface of the inner alveolar wall is always attempting to contract — much like the character exhibited in the way a raindrop holds itself together, or the way water holds itself together on the rim of a glass that is about to overflow. This contracting force exhibited by the watery inner alveolar surface makes for a naturally existing surface tension at the liquid-gas interface of the inner alveolar wall that inadvertently attempts to force air out of the alveoli through the bronchioles, thus promoting the collapse of the alveoli. To compensate for this phenomenon, the type 2 alveolar cells secrete alveolar fluid, which contains a substance known as surfactant. Surfactant lowers the surface tension of liquid-gas barrier and prevents the alveoli from collapsing upon expiration (exhaling).

Gas exchange in the alveoli

The exchange of oxygen and carbon dioxide occurs across the alveolar and capillary walls. The actual movement of oxygen and carbon dioxide across these membranes is accomplished by diffusion. Diffusion by definition means the movement of particles from an area of higher concentration of the particles to an area of lower concentration of the particles. Simply put, it means that a gas will move in the direction from where it is more concentrated to an area where it is less concentrated. A classic example of this is when you spray air freshener into a room. Upon spraying the can, the area immediately outside of the can is densely concentrated with air freshener particles and this is where you can smell the fragrance. Over time, however, you will eventually be able to smell the fragrance on the other side of the room. This is because the air freshener particles diffused across the room to areas of lower concentration.

The same principle is applied with the exchange of gases in the lungs where the concentration of these gases is measured in terms of what is known as their partial pressures. The partial pressure of a gas is simply a measure of its concentration in air or a liquid. Gases will always expand to fill the container they are in, whether it is a room or a microscopic-sized alveolus, and they always diffuse from areas of greater concentration or pressure to areas of lower concentration or pressure. The partial pressure of oxygen in the lungs is much higher than the partial pressure of oxygen in the blood that is passing through the alveolar capillaries. Remember, the blood that is circulating through the alveolar capillaries is blood that has just returned from the body after being used by the tissues, and it has very little oxygen remaining. Because the oxygen concentration of the blood in the alveolar capillaries is so low, a pressure gradient exists between the high oxygen concentration in the alveoli and the low oxygen concentration in the blood of the alveolar capillaries. Based on this concentration, or pressure gradient, oxygen diffuses from the alveoli of the lungs (the area of higher concentration or partial pressure) into the blood (the area of lower concentration or partial pressure).

The exact reverse is the case for carbon dioxide (CO_2). Carbon dioxide, the metabolic waste product of cellular metabolism, is continuously diffusing from the cells into the bloodstream. This provides for the concentration of carbon dioxide in the alveolar capillaries to be much higher than in the lungs, and therefore the pressure or concentration gradient of carbon dioxide is in the opposite direction of oxygen. Carbon dioxide, because its concentration is higher in the blood, diffuses from the alveolar capillaries (area of higher concentration of carbon dioxide) into the alveoli of the lungs (area of lower concentration of carbon dioxide) where it is then exhaled.

There are many sophisticated mechanisms in place that tightly monitor and control every detail of gas exchange between the lungs and the blood. The solubility of oxygen in water (or blood for that matter) is very low, therefore the vast majority (98 percent) of the oxygen that diffuses into the blood is transported by way of being bound to hemoglobin on red blood cells. The binding of oxygen to hemoglobin and its subsequent transport to the tissues is itself a very complex process that is under strict regulation. Although some carbon dioxide is also transported by hemoglobin (about 23 percent), the majority of carbon dioxide is transported in the form of bicarbonate. Bicarbonate (HCO_3^-) is the substance that is formed when carbon dioxide reacts with water, and this too is a very tightly controlled process so as to maintain the proper blood concentrations of carbon dioxide.

$$CO_2 + H_2O \rightleftharpoons H^+ + HCO_3^-$$

Figure 4 on the next page will help to visualize the exchange of oxygen and carbon dioxide at the alveolus–capillary interface.

Figure 4 **Illustration showing the exchange of oxygen and carbon dioxide between the alveolus (hollow space) and the surrounding capillary.**

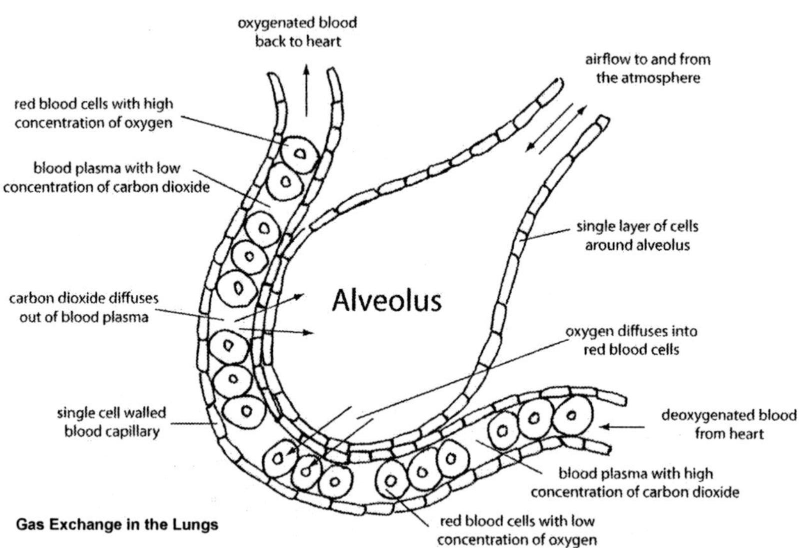

Perhaps seeing the concentrations of oxygen and carbon dioxide expressed in terms of their partial pressures will help reinforce the concept of gas exchange. The partial pressure of oxygen in alveolar air (the room air that is now down in the alveoli of the lungs) is 105 mm Hg. But the partial pressure of the oxygen in the blood within the alveolar capillaries (remember this is the deoxygenated blood from the pulmonary artery) is only 40 mm Hg. This is what we expect as there is more oxygen in the lungs than there is in the alveolar capillary blood at this point. Since gases flow from areas of higher partial pressures to areas of lower partial pressures, the oxygen flows from the alveoli of the lungs into the alveolar capillaries.

As for carbon dioxide, the same math holds true. The partial pressure of carbon dioxide in the alveoli is 40 mm Hg and the partial pressure of carbon dioxide in the blood within the alveolar capillaries is 45 mm Hg. This is consistent with what we expect to see as we know there is more carbon dioxide in the blood of the alveolar capillaries (blood from the pulmonary artery that contains the blood that was just returned to the heart after being used by the tissues) than in the alveoli of the lungs. Diffusion applies once again and carbon dioxide flows from the alveolar capillaries (area of higher concentration of carbon dioxide) into the alveoli of the lungs (area of lower concentration of carbon dioxide). Table 2 compares the differences in partial pressures of oxygen and carbon dioxide and their direction of flow across the alveolus-capillary interface.

Table 2

Relationship Between Partial Pressure and Direction of Gas Flow			
Gas	**Partial Pressure (mmHg)**		**Direction of Gas Flow**
	In lungs (alveoli)	**In deoxygenated blood** (alveolar capillaries — arterial side)	
Oxygen	105	40	From lungs into blood
Carbon Dioxide	40	45	From blood into lungs

Successful gas exchange and efficient transport of oxygen and carbon dioxide are critical to sustaining the immediate cellular requirements of life. Many of the problems that are associated with emphysema occur anatomically in the area that is local to where gas exchange occurs (the acinus). As the airway obstructions that are characteristic of COPD interfere with gas exchange, the task of keeping the airway open with minimal obstruction becomes an issue of primary importance. In one way or another, emphysema, chronic bronchitis, bronchiectasis, and the complications of infections and pneumonia all present their own unique ways of obstructing the airway and compromising the effectiveness of gas exchange. The task at hand is to teach you how to not only effectively address and lessen the severity of the immediate issues associated with an obstructed airway, but how to apply nutritional and natural health methods as part of a long-term effort to rebuild and maximize your health to the extent that you are able — one step at a time.

The mechanics of breathing and control of respiration

The mechanics of pulmonary ventilation (breathing) are accomplished through the actions of several muscle groups that are stimulated by nerve impulses that emanate from the respiratory center in the brain, namely the medulla and the pons. The main muscles involved with inspiration are the diaphragm, which is innervated by the phrenic nerve, and the external intercostals (muscles in between the ribs), which are innervated by the intercostal nerves. Accessory muscles used in inspiration are the sternocleidomastoid and the scalenes, both of which are in the neck.

The nervous system control of breathing is predominantly an involuntary (automatic) process, but can be voluntarily controlled as needed. The voluntary aspect is best evidenced in the interruption of breathing when you cough, or when you hold your breath for example. Overall regulation of breathing is controlled by neural and chemical reflex systems whose aim is to maintain the proper balance of oxygen delivery to, and carbon dioxide removal from, the tissues of the body.

The respiratory center in the brain stem is functionally divided into three areas with the main area being the medullary rhythmicity area located in the medulla oblongata. The basic automatic rhythm of respiration is set by inspiratory neurons in the medullary rhythmicity area. Neurons within this area spontaneously generate nerve impulses that initiate inspiration. These nerve impulses travel via the phrenic nerve to the diaphragm, and via the intercostal nerves to the external intercostal muscles causing contraction of these muscles, which results in inspiration. Contraction of the diaphragm and the external intercostal muscles increases the size of the thoracic cavity, and in so doing effectively creates a pressure differential whereby the pressure inside the chest cavity is now lower than the atmospheric pressure outside such that air flows into the lungs. Remember that gases flow in the direction of higher pressure to areas of lower pressure.

Nervous system regulation limits the time of the contraction of the diaphragm and the external intercostal muscles to just a couple of seconds, after which they relax until the next cycle. With the lungs now full of air, and the relaxation of the inspiratory muscles causing the size of the chest cavity to be reduced, you now have a situation where the pressure is higher inside the lungs — the opposite of before. As a result of the pressure differential being reversed, expiration occurs where air flows out of the lungs. Expiration during quiet breathing is normally passive as there are no muscular contractions involved. Expiration is accomplished through the elastic recoil of the lungs and the chest wall. During labored breathing, other rib muscles and abdominal muscles become involved to forcibly expel air. There are several other coordinating mechanisms that the body uses to either increase or decrease the rate of respiration. Changes in the pH of the blood, increased levels of carbon dioxide in the blood, elevated body temperature, or sudden severe pain will send messages to the respiratory center where the respiratory rate is adjusted to meet the current needs of the body.

Nerve supply to the lungs

The lungs are innervated (the nerve supply) by the anterior and posterior pulmonary plexuses (a network of intersecting nerves), which are mixed plexuses including sympathetic and parasympathetic fibers from the vagus nerve (cranial nerve X) and the sympathetic trunk. Sympathetic and parasympathetic nerve fibers are simply nerve fibers that are part of what is known as the autonomic, or involuntary nervous system. The autonomic nervous system (ANS) regulates vital bodily functions such as the activity of cardiac muscle, smooth muscle, and glands, and is controlled by the brain in a way that requires no conscious effort. ANS afferents (sensory fibers) carry pain fibers from the respiratory epithelium and stretch sensation from the bronchial tree and the alveolar sacs. ANS parasympathetic efferents (motor fibers) produce smooth muscle bronchoconstriction, vasodilation, and are secretomotor to the glands of the bronchial tree.   ANS sympathetic efferents cause smooth muscle bronchodilation, vasoconstriction, and are inhibitory to gland secretion.

Final remarks

The respiratory system is a marvelously complex system that maintains one of the most vital functions of the human body. There are literally endless volumes of material available that with varying degrees of complexity discuss the functioning of this remarkably intricate system. Inasmuch as the focus of this book is not on the nuances of respiratory anatomy or physiology, this chapter has presented sufficiently enough material to give you an overall familiarity of the basic structure and function of the respiratory system in order that you may have a greater appreciation for what is occurring in your own body. You will find this information useful in later chapters when you are learning about the various forms of COPD and natural/alternative therapeutics. You will have greater understanding of the particulars of your individual case, and moreover, you will appreciate how and why natural and alternative methods can be employed to help with your situation.

Chapter 2

Characteristics of Emphysema and COPD

Introduction

This chapter will introduce the pathology of emphysema and COPD. As one of the subdisciplines of medicine, pathology is the study of the causes, effects, and characteristics of disease. COPD is the blanket term that encompasses the conditions referred to by conventional medicine as emphysema, chronic bronchitis, bronchiectasis, and asthma. Although asthma is categorically under the umbrella of COPD, common medical parlance usually associates COPD with either emphysema or chronic bronchitis. As far as causes, progression, and therapeutic approaches are concerned, there are relationships that exist between emphysema and chronic bronchitis that do not exist between these two conditions and asthma. Bronchiectasis, although characteristically distinct from emphysema and chronic bronchitis, exhibits enough similarities to these two such that it is appropriate to include bronchiectasis in a discussion of COPD. This book will therefore confine its interests to emphysema, chronic bronchitis, and, to a lesser degree, bronchiectasis.

Emphysema and chronic bronchitis are predominantly characterized by dyspnea (shortness of breath) and chronic (ongoing or continually recurring) obstruction of the airflow through the lungs with reduced maximal expiratory flow during forced exhalation. Emphysema affects the acinus, whereas chronic bronchitis affects the bronchi and bronchioles; in many cases, individuals present with manifestations of both conditions because of the common underlying feature of cigarette smoking. With the exception of rare cases involving persons with an alpha 1 antitrypsin (alpha 1 AT) deficiency, a genetic condition that will be discussed later in this chapter, almost all cases of COPD involve persons who smoked at least a pack a day for twenty years or more.

The development of COPD is gradual, with the onset of the disease typically occurring in the forties. It is usually during the forties, after a lengthy history of smoking, that injury to the lungs becomes significant enough so as to enable the rendering of a diagnosis of COPD. It's not that you just "got COPD" in your forties — you were developing it ever since you started smoking in your teens or twenties. COPD is very insidious in this way insofar as it essentially hides itself from any real detection until it has already caused considerable damage. You may have experienced your share of colds or other respiratory infections throughout the years, but never anything ostensibly significant enough to suggest that serious respiratory disease was looming on the horizon. When you reach your forties, though, after twenty-plus years of smoking, and begin to experience the occasional shortness of breath and coughing of mucus that is often mistaken for being a cold or some other type of infection, the COPD that has been developing all these years has finally progressed enough such that the appropriate diagnostic tests will now enable a physician to make an accurate diagnosis of COPD.

Not all hope is lost, though. The key to having the greatest amount of success in minimizing any further progression is to stop smoking and begin addressing your health as soon as you are first diagnosed. The problem with many people who have been diagnosed with COPD in their forties is that they ignore the seriousness of their diagnosis. My own father is a prime example. He was diagnosed in his forties but continued to smoke for another twenty-five years until he was finally diagnosed with laryngeal cancer and had to have his larynx surgically removed, leaving him to breathe through a stoma in his neck. By this time his COPD was also quite severe; it was only at this point that he completely stopped smoking and, along with conventional medicine, began to utilize nutritional methods and natural medicine in an effort to rebuild his health. The upside to his story is that he celebrated his eighty-second birthday this year and is doing relatively well, all things considered.

Your take-home lesson from this is to not delay in reestablishing your health. It has been said that an ounce of prevention is better than a pound of cure, and that could not be any truer than in the case of COPD. Your best prevention would have been to have never started to smoke in the first place; however, that is essentially water under the bridge at this point. You are now at a crossroads as far as your health is concerned; so make the best decision for yourself and begin the process of rebuilding your health today. Give yourself every benefit of the doubt that you can and begin taking the appropriate measures to regain your health. I cannot emphasize enough that the earlier you begin to employ natural health practices, the better off you will be.

Any therapeutic method, whether it is conventional, natural, or alternative, will always have its limitations, and oftentimes those limitations are based upon how far a condition has progressed by the time intervention begins. Natural medicine can be helpful at any stage of progression of an illness, but the earlier you begin to employ natural health practices, the greater overall benefit you will eventually realize in your life. Remember that you did not develop COPD overnight. It took years to take effect on your body. By the same token, you will not rebuild your health overnight. But if you start now, you'll afford yourself the best possible chance to build up your health so that in the coming years, and for the rest of your life for that matter, you'll have developed a health-promoting lifestyle rather than a life of succumbing to disease.

Conventional diagnostic methods

Because the onset of COPD is gradual, and almost always related to a history of smoking, its diagnosis is often not a surprise, although that doesn't make it any easier to digest. Your diagnosis of COPD could have come as a result of a routine visit to your physician's office. Perhaps your visit to the ER or your physician's office came as a result of having what you thought was a respiratory infection or a cold that had become bothersome enough that it needed professional attention. In either case, the physician's examination resulted in certain findings that led him or her to follow up with additional tests that ultimately revealed that the COPD that had been developing for years had now begun to manifest itself symptomatically.

There are a variety of symptoms that can be experienced that are the cardinal signs of COPD. These symptoms could also be indicative of problems other than COPD, but nonetheless, if you are experiencing the following symptoms, it is time to get yourself evaluated by your physician.

<u>COPD Symptoms</u>

Dyspnea (shortness of breath) — Dyspnea may occur as a result of exertion, but it may also occur while at rest. Dyspnea commonly occurs when it becomes harder to breathe due to decreased elasticity of the lungs.

Cough — A cough is a normal protective reflex that can be brought about by mechanical, chemical, or inflammatory factors. It is the most common symptom of respiratory disease and a prominent sign of chronic bronchitis. An unexplainable cough lasting longer than two or three weeks definitely needs to be evaluated by a physician.

Sputum (mucus) — Excessive mucus that gradually increases over the years is a hallmark for chronic bronchitis and bronchiectasis. Yellow sputum is indicative of an infection. Green sputum, which is indicative of stagnant pus, and often foul smelling, is commonly associated with bronchiectasis.

Hemoptysis (coughing up blood) — Coughing up blood from the respiratory tract can be indicative of a very serious problem and should be evaluated as soon as possible. Pneumonia, bronchiectasis, tuberculosis, and lung cancer are some of the causes of having blood in the sputum. If you experience blood in your sputum, you need to see your physician at once.

Digital clubbing — Digital clubbing is a phenomenon whereby the angle between the nail and the finger is increased and the fingers take on a drumstick appearance. The appearance of digital clubbing is not understood; however, it has been clearly established that in approximately 75 percent of the time that digital clubbing is present, it is due to respiratory disease, although not necessarily COPD.

Chest pain — Chest pain can result from a myriad of reasons, but when it relates to respiratory disease, it is often due to inflammation of the parietal pleura. In any case, chest pain should always be evaluated by a physician.

Cyanosis — Cyanosis is when the skin and mucous membranes (mainly on the face, lips, and earlobes) take on a bluish discoloration because there is an excess of deoxygenated hemoglobin in the blood. Cyanosis can be indicative of insufficient oxygenation of the blood and needs to be evaluated by a physician to determine its exact cause.

In order to evaluate your symptoms, your physician will need to study your past medical history and conduct a thorough physical examination. Various blood tests and other diagnostic procedures will also be used in order to conclusively confirm a diagnosis of COPD. Some of the tests or procedures that may be used to confirm COPD are as follows:

<u>COPD Diagnostic Tests</u>

Radiological procedures — The chest x-ray is often one of the studies used to rule out any other lung diseases besides COPD, as the chest x-ray itself is rather imprecise in determining COPD unless the COPD is quite severe. A CT scan may provide more accuracy in diagnosing COPD, although some abnormal lung anatomy still may not be detected.

Arterial blood gases — Arterial blood is able to yield very useful information that cannot be obtained from venous blood. Arterial blood gases are usually obtained from blood drawn from the radial artery in the wrist. Arterial blood is measured to determine PaO_2 (the partial pressure of oxygen, or the concentration of oxygen in the arterial blood), SaO_2 (the percentage of hemoglobin saturated with oxygen in the arterial blood), and $PaCO_2$ (the partial pressure of carbon dioxide, or the concentration of carbon dioxide in the arterial blood). Abnormally low values of PaO_2 are referred to as hypoxemia, and it often indicates hypoxia (inadequate amounts of oxygen in the tissues). Elevated values of $PaCO_2$ are referred to as hypercapnia. This often occurs because COPD patients tend to retain carbon dioxide as a result of their inability to ventilate completely. This is an area of particular concern as COPD patients can become tolerant of the elevated carbon dioxide levels such that hypoxia becomes the principal drive for respiration. Under these circumstances, if the patient is being given supplemental oxygen, the amount of oxygen being given must be carefully controlled. If the patient is given too high a concentration of oxygen, a commensurate amount of carbon dioxide will be produced, yet the carbon dioxide will be retained (hypercapnia) due to their decreased ventilation status. This increase of retained carbon dioxide will cause respiratory acidosis, which is indicated by a marked lowering of the pH of the blood, and will lead to dire consequences if not corrected. Arterial blood, therefore, is also used to determine the pH of the blood (the hydrogen ion concentration, or the acid/base character of the blood), and the concentration of HCO_3^- (bicarbonate, or the blood buffering system).

Oximetry (pulse ox) — This is the plastic clip that is placed on your fingertip in the hospital or the doctor's office that gives a reasonably accurate measurement of the oxygenation of the blood. It is not as accurate as the information derived from an arterial blood gas; however, it is practical in that it can be used to measure the oxygenation of the blood during activity or during sleep.

Alpha 1 antitrypsin level — This is a simple blood test to determine if you have the genetically inherited form of emphysema due to an alpha 1 AT deficiency.

Pulmonary function tests — There are generally four different aspects of pulmonary function testing. They are spirometry, post-bronchodilator spirometry, lung volume testing, and diffusion capacity.

Spirometry — This test measures the amount of air entering and exiting the lungs and is the most reliable way of determining reversible airway obstruction. To perform the test, a patient inhales as deeply as possible, and then exhales as forcefully and rapidly as possible into the spirometry machine until they can exhale no more. The test yields several measurements; however, the most commonly used measurements used in determining the presence of COPD are the FEV_1 (forced expiratory volume after 1 second), and the FVC (forced vital capacity). Individuals with COPD typically show a reduction in the amount of air exhaled (FVC) compared to individuals with healthy lungs. COPD patients also show a reduction in the amount of air exhaled during the initial first second of exhalation (FEV_1), and the reduction in FEV_1 is to a greater degree than the FVC reduction. This means that COPD patients not only exhale less, but they exhale significantly less during the first second of exhalation. Individuals with healthy lungs usually exhale upwards of 75 percent of the air they inhaled during the first second of exhalation, but in persons with COPD that percentage is much lower.

Post–bronchodilator spirometry — Post-bronchodilator spirometry utilizes the same process that is used for regular spirometry, except that it is performed after the patient has been given a bronchodilator, such as albuterol. If there is improvement in the FEV_1, it indicates that the airways are responsive to the drug, and that it may be useful in the management of the airway obstruction.

Lung volume testing — Lung volume testing reveals very useful information in the diagnosis of emphysema. Two important measurements obtained from lung volume testing are residual volume (RV), and total lung capacity (TLC). A high TLC indicates hyperinflation (overinflation) of the lungs, and a high RV indicates that air is being trapped in the lungs. High values for TLC and RV are indicative of emphysema.

Diffusion capacity — This test measures how much gas is transferred from the alveoli into the capillaries. A very small and safe amount of carbon monoxide is inhaled, and then the blood is tested to see how much carbon monoxide diffused from the lungs into the bloodstream. A reduced diffusion capacity is indicative of emphysema. Table 3 provides a summary of the abbreviations used in some of the various diagnostic tests for COPD.

Table 3

Abbreviations Used in Some of the Various Diagnostic Tests for COPD

PaO_2 The partial pressure (concentration) of oxygen in arterial blood.

SaO_2 The percentage of hemoglobin saturated with oxygen in arterial blood.

$PaCO_2$ The partial pressure (concentration) of carbon dioxide in arterial blood.

FEV_1 Forced expiratory volume in one second. This is the amount of air exhaled in one second after maximal inhalation.

FVC   Forced vital capacity. This is the maximal amount of air exhaled after maximal inhalation.

RV   Residual volume. This is the amount of air left in the lungs after a forced exhalation.

TLC   Total lung capacity. This is the amount of air that can be contained in the lungs after maximal inhalation.

DLCO   Diffusion capacity of the lungs for carbon monoxide.

Emphysema — overview

Emphysema is defined as the abnormal and permanent enlargement of the airspaces (alveoli) distal to the terminal bronchioles. Respiratory bronchioles in affected acini are usually narrower and convoluted, and their walls have experienced various degrees of atrophy. Pulmonary fibrosis (the proliferation of fibrous connective tissue) is usually not seen with emphysema proper; however, the formation of scar tissue in the connective tissue of the lungs is usually a consequence of inflammation, or irritation caused by bronchopneumonia, which is often an ongoing complication in persons with COPD. The abnormal enlargement of the airspaces is brought about as a result of the collapse of the alveolar wall due to the destruction of elastin fibers that are contained within the wall. Recall that alveoli are the single-cell-layered airspaces (gas bubbles), surrounded by capillaries, where gas exchange occurs. Recall as well that in addition to comprising the alveolar sacs, alveoli are also present along the respiratory bronchioles. The precise location along the acinus of collapsed walls is in large part the determining factor in identifying what type of emphysema is present, and these different types will be discussed later in the chapter, but for now, let us further explore the architecture of the acinus and understand what is meant by the destruction or collapse of the alveolar wall.

Earlier in chapter 1 the metaphor of a cluster of grapes was used to paint a picture of the acinus. Think of that metaphor again, except now consider a few changes and additions that must be made in order to further clarify what occurs in the case of emphysema. To begin with, the stems and the grapes themselves must be imagined as hollow. The individual grapes (alveoli) do not exist completely independent of one another. They are immediately adjacent to one another, separated only by a fine septum called the interalveolar septum (a matrix consisting of connective tissue fibers and capillaries), and are interconnected to each other by what are known as Pores of Kohn. These pores are essentially holes that exist between the alveoli (grapes) that allow for the complete ventilation of air throughout the acinus. It is essential to realize that there is no truly free space between alveoli. They are always surrounded by a matrix of connective tissue fibers and capillaries — the interalveolar septum. Another useful metaphor at this point to elaborate upon the architecture of the acinus is to picture a building full of empty rooms with no windows.

Imagine entering a building that immediately leads you down a single main hallway. This main hallway is synonymous with a respiratory bronchiole. There are a few rooms (alveoli) along this hallway, all of which have an archway opening with no true door attached. Now you take a turn and go down a secondary hallway. This secondary hallway is synonymous with an alveolar duct, and there are numerous rooms along this hallway. None of these rooms has a door either, only an archway space where a door would be. Imagine that as you enter any particular room in this secondary hallway, you find another archway in that room that leads to yet another room. Imagine this pattern continuing on so as to eventually become an elaborate labyrinth. This labyrinth is synonymous with an alveolar sac, where the rooms that are interconnected by archways within the labyrinth are the alveoli, and the internal archways themselves are the Pores of Kohn. Each one of the initial doorways in the secondary hallway (alveolar duct) leads to its own labyrinth of rooms (alveolar sacs). The important thing to visualize is that once a room is entered into from the secondary hallway (the alveolar duct), there are no more hallways separating individual rooms (the alveoli) that lie deeper within that particular labyrinth (the alveolar sac), only the archways (Pores of Kohn).

Consider hypothetically that in any one particular labyrinth (alveolar sac) there are twenty rooms (twenty alveoli) interconnected by archways (Pores of Kohn). Consider now the walls of each of the rooms. Although the archways interconnect the rooms, the walls are what separate the rooms from each other. The surface of the walls (the sheetrock) represents the alveolar wall, and the inside of the walls (the studs, plumbing, etc.) represents the interalveolar septum; however, for all practical purposes the alveolar wall and the interalveolar septum can be thought of as a continuous structure. In anatomical language, a septum is a partition or wall that separates two structures. In reality, the interalveolar septum is the structure that separates the alveoli. In our grape cluster metaphor, the septum would be the matrix that surrounds and coats all the grapes (alveoli). Within that matrix are contained fine collagen and elastin fibers, which are interlaced amongst a vast capillary network. In terms of the rooms/walls metaphor, the studs within the walls represent the matrix of collagen and elastin fibers, and the plumbing within the walls represents the capillary network.

To complete this overview of the destruction of the alveolar wall using the room metaphor, remember that the hallways and rooms must all be seen as empty, and whose only purpose is to facilitate the circulation of air. As air travels down the main hallway (respiratory bronchiole) on into the secondary hallway (alveolar duct), the air finds itself ultimately being circulated throughout the rooms (alveoli) as well. All is well as long as clean air is the only thing being circulated throughout this system. When you start circulating cigarette smoke or other noxious substances throughout this system, you begin to have problems. Over time the chemicals in the smoke will wear down the walls, and eventually the walls will collapse and break.

Each room has its dimensions, which, when calculated, would determine the surface area of that room (the available area for gas exchange). The sum of the surface areas of all the rooms within any particular labyrinth would give the total surface area of the labyrinth. When a wall is destroyed, you lose the surface area of that wall. Instead of having two rooms separated by a wall, there is now one big room without a dividing wall, which effectively amounts to a permanently enlarged airspace. When this damage happens in multiple rooms throughout the labyrinth, you have a serious problem because now many rooms (alveoli/airspaces) have been enlarged, resulting in a significant overall compromise of the available surface area for gas exchange. Figures 5 and 6 show the differences between normal and emphysematous alveoli.

Figure 5 **Illustration of an electron micrograph of normal alveoli. Grayish regions are the alveoli, darker regions are the alveolar ducts. Note the interalveolar septa (the thicker white areas within the grayish regions that serve as the borders, or walls, that separate the alveoli).**

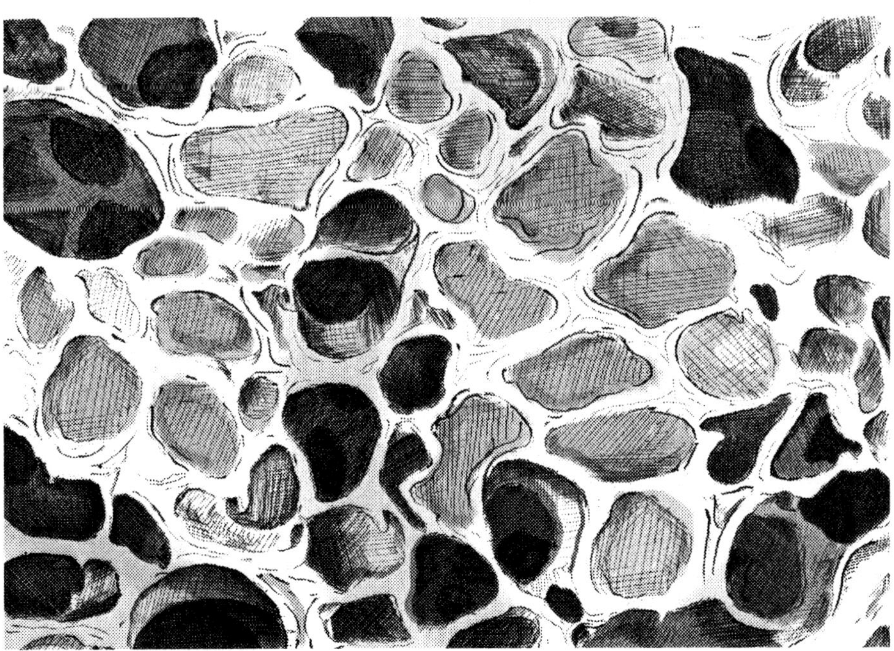

***Figure* 6 Illustration of an electron micrograph of emphysematous alveoli at the same magnification as figure 5. Note the loss of interalveolar septa (destroyed walls), and enlarged alveolar spaces.**

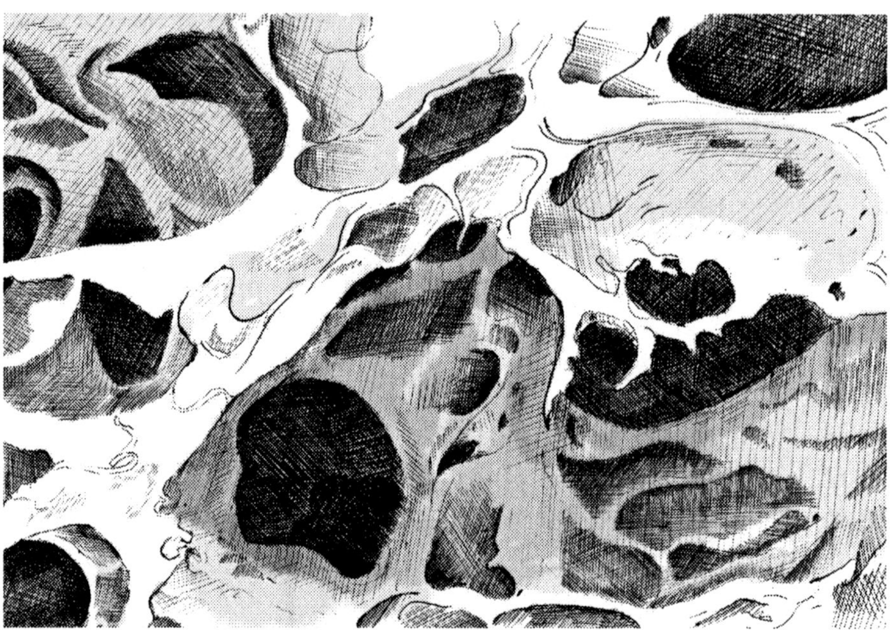

This is the central issue of emphysema: the collapse of the alveolar walls that leads to abnormal and permanent enlargement of the airspaces. Loss of the walls not only creates enlarged airspaces, but it also means a loss of surface area for the exchange of carbon dioxide and oxygen, as well as a lessening of the elasticity of the lungs.

Destruction of the walls also leads to disruptions in certain structural arrangements of the lungs that are necessary in maintaining unobstructed, open airways (mainly terminal and respiratory bronchioles). There are several forces that work together to ensure that these microscopic-sized airways are always kept maximally open. One such force is radial traction, which is essentially a force exerted through the lung tissue surrounding a bronchiole that helps to hold the bronchiole open. When the alveolar walls are destroyed, you not only have the consequent enlargement of the airspaces, but you also have a disruption in the overall structural arrangement of the local lung tissue. With this disruption in structure, the lung tissue surrounding a bronchiole becomes less effective at exerting the radial traction necessary to help keep the airway (bronchiole) open. This results in a potential lessening of the diameter of the particular airway (bronchiole), which amounts to being an obstruction.

Emphysema — pathogenesis

To the extent that cigarette smoking is a well-established pathogenic factor and the main causative agent in emphysema, it is possible for other inhaled noxious substances to produce the pathological picture of emphysema. The exact mechanism of how inhaled noxious chemicals destroy the alveolar wall is still not yet completely understood, and the determination of this mechanism remains an area of current research. However, it is presently believed that the collapse of the alveolar wall is due to a protease–anti-protease imbalance that results in the enzymatic destruction of the elastic fibers (elastin) that exist within the alveolar wall, the area specifically referred to as the interalveolar septum.

Elastin is a protein and is the principal molecule that comprises the elastic fibers within the interalveolar septum. A protease is an enzyme that acts as a catalyst in the breakdown of a protein. The protease in question is known as neutrophil lysosomal elastase. Alpha 1 AT, a protein that is produced in the liver and found in the blood, tissue fluids, and macrophages, acts in a way so as to inhibit the action of elastase.

It appears that the chemicals in cigarette smoke stimulate the accumulation of macrophages and neutrophils in the lung. A neutrophil is a granular white blood cell that is a normal part of the immune system whose job is to protect the body either through phagocytosis (engulfing of foreign substances) or proteolysis (the breaking down of proteins). Macrophages and neutrophils are normally present as part of the defense mechanism of the lungs; however, evidence seems to indicate that cigarette smoke stimulates alveolar macrophages to release neutrophil chemotactic factors, which are simply molecules that cause the increased recruitment of neutrophils into the lung. Nicotine itself is chemotactic for (attracts) neutrophils, and the very presence of nicotine will cause increased recruitment of neutrophils into the lungs. This excessive recruitment of neutrophils into the lungs creates an imbalance that leads to the destruction of the interalveolar septum. Upon reaching the lungs, neutrophils escape from capillary circulation and enter into the matrix of the interalveolar septum by way of a process known as diapedesis. Diapedesis is the mechanism by which red or white blood cells are passed through — essentially oozed through — the wall of the blood vessel that contains them without damaging the vessel itself.

Once in the interalveolar septum, neutrophils release proteases (enzymes) that in turn degrade proteins. Specifically, in this case, the neutrophil releases lysosomal elastase, and neutrophil elastase is very capable of digesting the elastin in the interalveolar septum. Although both macrophages and neutrophils release elastase, it is believed that neutrophil elastase plays a more important role in the destruction of elastin in the alveolar wall. Neutrophil elastase is also capable of destroying type IV collagen, another important molecule that contributes to the structure of the alveolar wall. Neutrophils and alveolar macrophages also release a messenger molecule known as leukotriene B_4, and leukotriene B_4 acts as a signal to recruit more neutrophils. This further contributes to the inflammation and destruction of the interalveolar septum. Leukotrienes will be discussed in more detail beginning in chapter 3.

Under normal circumstances, meaning in the absence of repeated exposure to cigarette smoke or other noxious chemicals, alpha 1 AT would diffuse from the capillary circulation into the interalveolar septum and keep the activity of neutrophil elastase at bay. The problem, though, is that stimulated neutrophils also release oxygen free radicals, and oxygen free radicals inhibit the activity of alpha 1 AT. Alpha 1 AT therefore cannot keep the activity of neutrophil elastase at bay. With alpha 1 AT being "tied up," so to speak, it is unable to stop neutrophil elastase from destroying the elastin within the alveolar wall.

Like all proteins, alpha 1 AT is a long chain of amino acid molecules linked together. The important amino acid in this long chain is methionine 358. Alpha 1 AT normally inhibits the activity of neutrophil elastase by attaching its methionine 358 section nearly irreversibly to the active portion of elastase, and in so doing it alters the structure of elastase such that elastase loses its enzymatic ability to digest elastin. However, as a consequence of the oxidants in cigarette smoke, as well as neutrophils also releasing oxygen free radicals into the area, alpha 1 AT ends up reacting with these oxidants or oxygen free radicals rather than to elastase. Oxidants and oxygen free radicals are very reactive species that are capable of reacting indiscriminately with other molecules. These reactive species oxidize the methionine 358 of the alpha 1 AT. This means that the oxidants or the oxygen free radicals react with the methionine 358 and attach oxygen to the methionine 358 section of the alpha 1 AT. In so doing, it converts the methionine into methionine sulfoxide, and that alters the structure of alpha 1 AT such that it can no longer recognize neutrophil elastase. When alpha 1 AT can no longer recognize elastase, it cannot inhibit the activity of elastase, which is to say that alpha 1 AT loses its ability to prevent elastase from destroying elastin. With the consequent destruction of elastin, the alveolar wall collapses, the airspaces become enlarged, and the lungs lose elasticity. Table 4 summarizes the events leading to the destruction of the interalveolar septum, and hence the alveolar wall.

Table 4

Summary of the Sequence of Events in the Destruction of the Alveolar Wall

1. The acinus is repeatedly exposed to cigarette smoke or other noxious chemicals.
2. Continuous exposure to smoke, etc. induces excessive recruitment of macrophages and neutrophils into the lung.
   A. Macrophages release neutrophil chemotactic factors, which cause recruitment of neutrophils into the lung.
   B. Nicotine itself, as a chemotactic agent for neutrophils, causes recruitment of neutrophils into the lung.
3. Upon entering the lung, neutrophils escape capillary circulation and find their way into the interalveolar septum through the process of diapedesis.
4. Once in the interalveolar septum, neutrophils release lysosomal elastase, an enzyme that degrades elastin, the principal component of the elastic fibers within the interalveolar septum. Neutrophils can also perpetuate their own existence through their release of the molecular messenger leukotriene B_4.
5. Alpha 1 antitrypsin, a protein that would normally inhibit the action of neutrophil elastase, is rendered ineffective due it being tied up by reactive oxygen free radicals released from neutrophils as well as oxidants in cigarette smoke.
6. As a result of elastin in the interalveolar septum being degraded by neutrophil elastase, the alveolar wall collapses, resulting in permanent, abnormal enlargement of the airspaces, and a lessening of the elasticity of the lungs.

Emphysema — alpha 1 antitrypsin deficiency

Greater than 80 percent of all COPD cases are directly related to cigarette smoking. Approximately 10–15 percent of cases are non-smoking related where the condition of COPD results from long-term continual exposure to noxious irritants other than cigarette smoke. A small percentage of emphysema cases, approximately 2–5 percent, are caused by what is known as an alpha 1 antitrypsin (alpha 1 AT) deficiency. The manifestation of emphysema in this small group is not solely due to any exposure to cigarette smoke or chemical irritants, but rather because the body itself failed to make alpha 1 AT correctly. Recall that the job of alpha 1 AT is to stop neutrophil elastase from destroying elastin in the alveolar wall. To the extent that oxygen free radicals from cigarette smoke and neutrophils alter the structure of alpha 1 AT so as to render it ineffective in inhibiting elastase, when the body fails to make alpha 1 AT correctly due to a genetic defect, this becomes the second means by which alpha 1 AT is rendered ineffective. As a result, protection against the destructive action of neutrophil elastase is greatly diminished.

As discussed in the previous section, alpha 1 AT is a protein made predominantly by the cells of the liver and then released into the blood circulation. Proteins are made up of molecules that are known as amino acids. Amino acids are a collection of about twenty different molecules that when assembled together into very specific arrangements become functional proteins. Some of these amino acids are synthesized by your body, whereas others have to be derived through the food you eat. Protein that you acquire through the food that you eat, however, is not in a form that is usable by your body. When you eat protein-containing foods, the protein is digested and broken up into amino acid components. The cells of the body then need to arrange and assemble those amino acid components in specific sequences in order for them to become functional proteins that the body can then utilize. As with all proteins, the instructions for the assembly of these amino acids are contained within the DNA (deoxyribonucleic acid) that is housed within the nuclei of the cells of the body.

DNA contains the instructions to make all the necessary proteins for the body. DNA is merely a strand of code molecules that serves as the template for protein manufacturing. DNA never leaves the nucleus of the cell. Since proteins are actually assembled in another part of the cell called the cytoplasm, there needs to be a way to get the instructions from the DNA out of the nucleus and into the cytoplasm of the cell. The cell accomplishes this task by having the DNA transcribe its code into another strand of code known as messenger RNA (ribonucleic acid). The strand of mRNA will contain the same sequence of code (instructions) as the original DNA. The mRNA is able to leave the nucleus and travel into the cytoplasm where it can then be used as the coding template to make a protein.

The mRNA template (instructional code sequence) is translated very specifically in order to make a protein. If there is any alteration in the sequence of the code, then the protein will not get made correctly. In order for alpha 1 AT to be made properly, a series of amino acids must be assembled together in a very specific sequence. The sequence of how the amino acids are assembled is dictated by the code within the mRNA. For various different reasons, including genetic inheritance, the sequence of the code can become altered (mutated). An entire code of instructions that consists of hundreds of molecules within the mRNA template can be completely ruined by mutating just one molecule of code. This is the case with an alpha 1 AT deficiency. The genetic code that serves as the template to assemble alpha 1 AT is altered by just one molecule.   The result is that you end up making a defective protein that does not possess the ability to carry out the functions that alpha 1 AT should normally be able to perform, mainly the ability to inhibit the activity of neutrophil elastase. This is why these types of emphysema patients are referred to as alpha 1 AT deficient. As a result of a genetic predisposition, these patients do not have optimally functional alpha 1 AT.

Despite its being genetically inherited from birth, many individuals with an alpha 1 AT deficiency who are lifelong nonsmokers do not develop emphysema. If you have genetically inherited alpha 1 AT deficiency, you are at much greater risk for developing emphysema; however, the evidence strongly indicates that for individuals who are genetically deficient for alpha 1 AT, cigarette smoking still remains the single most important cofactor in the actual development of emphysema. What this means is that if you have a genetically inherited deficiency of alpha 1 AT, and you never smoke cigarettes, you may not develop emphysema to any extent that becomes clinically significant. If, however, you have a genetically inherited deficiency of alpha 1 AT, and you do smoke cigarettes, you will in all likelihood not only develop emphysema, but you will develop it at a much earlier age and experience it much more severely due to your deficiency of alpha 1 AT.

These findings seem to be consistent with current understanding regarding the destruction of the alveolar wall. Even though an individual may have a genetically inherited deficiency of alpha 1 AT, in the absence of cigarette smoking, there is no significant accumulation of neutrophils into the lung. With no significant accumulation of neutrophils into the lung, there is no appreciable amount of elastase in the lung, either. In a scenario such as this, a deficiency of alpha 1 AT is not missed as much, as there is less need for it because the threat of damage due to elastase is minimal. But if you introduce a history of cigarette smoking into this scenario, you now have a situation where there is continuous recruitment of neutrophils into the lungs that in turn release their destructive elastase, and because of a genetic deficiency, you have no functional alpha 1 AT to act as an inhibitor of the elastase. You now have a scenario that is inviting disaster. At the end of the day, however, whether or not you are alpha 1 AT deficient seems not to be the major factor in developing emphysema. The crux of the situation still seems to lie in whether or not you smoked.

Besides not being able to adequately inhibit neutrophil elastase in the alveolar wall, improperly made alpha 1 AT can cause other significant problems. Aberrant alpha 1 AT has other complications associated with it that make it difficult to exit the cells of the liver. In adults, the aberrant alpha 1 AT that remains in the liver can lead to cirrhosis of the liver. With children, although alpha 1 AT deficiency rarely ever leads to emphysema, many of them will develop chronic liver disease ranging from neonatal hepatitis to progressive cirrhosis while still in infancy. For these reasons, anyone who has a diagnosis of alpha 1 AT deficiency should, at a minimum, be on a daily regime of milk thistle. More will be said about milk thistle in chapters 3 and 5.

Alpha 1 AT deficiency can be diagnosed with a simple blood test. Anyone who has a history of cigarette smoking should be tested for alpha 1 AT deficiency. Nonsmokers who begin to develop symptoms that are part of the classic picture for COPD should also be tested. Alpha

1 AT deficiency is treated with weekly I.V. administration of alpha 1 AT derived from human blood. Currently this treatment is only available to patients who meet the criteria of having low enough blood levels of alpha 1 AT and who also have fully manifested emphysema.

Emphysema — classifications

Earlier in this chapter it is stated that the precise location along the acinus of the collapsed walls is in large part the determining factor in identifying what type of emphysema is present. Although emphysema is defined as the abnormal and permanent enlargement of the airspaces, the exact location of where this is occurring within the acinus leads to the classification of four major types of emphysema.

Centrilobular emphysema — Centrilobular, or centriacinar emphysema, is the most common type of emphysema. It involves primarily the respiratory bronchioles and their alveoli. The alveoli within the alveolar sacs are usually less involved. This is the type of emphysema seen most often in cigarette smokers, and it predominantly affects the upper lobes of the lung, in the area of the lung closest to the shoulders. There is usually inflammation associated with the bronchi, bronchioles, and the interalveolar septum. Because of the strong causal link to cigarette smoking, this form of emphysema is often seen in combination with chronic bronchitis.

Panlobular emphysema — Panlobular, or panacinar emphysema, is the type of emphysema most often associated with alpha 1 AT deficiency. Panlobular emphysema tends to occur more often in the lower zones of the lung and is most severe at the base of the lung. In panlobular emphysema the entire acinus is affected, and uniform enlargement of the airspaces is present from the respiratory bronchiole all the way to the distal alveoli. In cases of panlobular emphysema where the damage is extensive, there is marked reduction in the gas exchange surface (alveoli-capillary interface) as well as a reduction in the elastic recoil properties of the lungs.

Paraseptal emphysema — Paraseptal, or distal acinar emphysema, predominantly affects the most distal part of the acinus, the alveolar sacs and alveoli. It is more pronounced at the margins of the lobules, and in areas near the pleura, and tends to occur next to areas that have been subjected to fibrosis or scarring. This type of emphysema is usually more severe in the upper regions of the lungs and can be the cause of spontaneous pneumothorax, which is a condition where air or gas enters into the pleural space and causes the lung to collapse.

Irregular emphysema — Irregular emphysema is so called because it lacks any definable regularity regarding the part of the acinus that is involved. What is understood, though, is that this type of emphysema is always associated with scarring.

Bullae are enlarged airspaces that are greater than 1 cm in diameter and can be present with any of the four types of emphysema. They occupy areas right next to the visceral pleura, usually near the apex (top) of the lungs. When these localized areas are especially prominent, the condition is sometimes referred to as bullous emphysema. Bullous emphysema presents its own unique set of concerns due to the potential size of the bullae and their potential for rupture. Bullae that become large enough can compromise breathing by compressing healthy lung tissue that is adjacent to the bullae. A ruptured bulla can give rise to a pneumothorax.

Chronic bronchitis — overview and pathogenesis

Chronic bronchitis is characterized by the excessive production of mucus in the bronchi, along with a productive cough, not caused by any other reason, that is present on most days for at least three months per year over a period of two consecutive years. As with emphysema, the main causative agent in the development of chronic bronchitis is cigarette smoking, although other inhaled toxic substances and recurrent respiratory infections can also bring about its development.

Sustained exposure and continuous irritation from cigarette smoke leads to chronic inflammation as well as morphological (physical structure) changes in the cells lining the respiratory tract. Recall from chapter 1 the mucous-secreting goblet cells that are part of the respiratory epithelium in the bronchi and bronchioles. Recall also that throughout the trachea and bronchi are glands known as submucosal mucous-secreting glands. It is currently believed that repeated exposure to the chemical toxins in cigarette smoke causes hypertrophy and hyperplasia of the submucosal mucous-secreting glands, which in turn leads to hypersecretion (excessive secretion) of mucus in the bronchi. Hypertrophy of the submucosal glands means that these glands have become enlarged. These glands become enlarged because the cells that comprise them have become enlarged due to constant irritation from cigarette smoke. Hyperplasia, on the other hand, refers to an actual increase in the number of gland cells, also believed to be due to irritation from cigarette smoke toxins. You essentially end up having an overabundance of larger-than-normal submucosal mucous-secreting glands, which results in the oversecretion of mucus into the airway. This oversecretion of mucus clogs the airway, often as mucus plugs, and the mucus itself becomes an obstruction in the airway. Cigarette smoke also impairs the sweeping motion of cilia on the respiratory epithelium, which further complicates the obstructive process, as the bronchial passages, which are now faced with even more mucus, are less able to clear themselves.

Evidence also suggests that chronic inflammatory changes occur in the smaller airways, mainly secondary and tertiary bronchi, and the portion of the bronchioles that still contains goblet cells. It appears that as chronic bronchitis and its accompanying inflammation persist, there is a consequent increase in the number of mucous-secreting goblet cells that are found amongst the epithelial cells in these smaller airways. With an increased number of goblet cells, there is excessive mucus production, and oversecretion of this mucus ends up clogging and obstructing these smaller airways.

Besides obstructing the airways, excessive mucus production leads to another problem that can seriously complicate the therapeutic management of COPD. Excessive mucus serves as a breeding ground for bacterial growth, which in turn becomes one of the main reasons why COPD patients often experience recurrent respiratory infections. Acute episodes of infection are accompanied by inflammation and further mucus production, which make for a vicious cycle that becomes increasingly difficult to manage as COPD continues to progress. The nutritional and natural health approaches to reducing inflammation so as to limit mucus production and prevent infections are major areas of concern that will be given significant attention in the subsequent chapters of this book.

Chronic bronchitis — inflammation

Although oversecretion of mucus and prevention of infection are areas of great concern, addressing the underlying issue of inflammation that resulted from the constant irritation by cigarette smoke and/or recurrent infections is of primary importance. Treating hypersecretion of mucus and exacerbations due to infections will always remain an uphill battle if the underlying inflammation is not concurrently addressed.

Inflammation can be acute or chronic. The acute inflammatory response is the normal initial response by the immune system when the body is subjected to a harmful insult (an invading infection or toxic agent). When the body is subjected to an insult, the acute inflammatory response occurs whereby white blood cells are summoned to the affected tissue to protect that tissue from the insult. As white blood cells infiltrate (move into) the tissue as part of the body's normal response to defend itself against the insult, a series of very complicated cellular and molecular events ensues as part of the inflammatory process. Ultimately the insult is eradicated, tissue is subsequently healed, and the acute inflammatory response ceases. If, however, the insult is continuous, or the healing process is interfered with, the acute inflammatory response will not cease. White blood cells will continue to maintain their presence in the affected tissue, and the acute inflammation will eventually progress to chronic inflammation.

There are several different types of white blood cells involved in the inflammatory process, as well as many other molecules that act as mediators (messengers) of the inflammatory process. Some of the main white blood cells involved in the inflammatory process associated with chronic bronchitis are lymphocytes, eosinophils, macrophages, and neutrophils. Some of the major classes of mediator molecules that act as messengers between these cells are leukotrienes, cytokines, and chemokines.

Chronic inflammation does not have to arise from acute inflammation; it often develops quite insidiously without any apparent symptoms. This is how the chronic inflammation associated with chronic bronchitis is believed to develop. In chronic bronchitis you have a situation where low-grade, yet active, inflammation exists as a consequence of the constant irritation from cigarette smoke, and it continues to develop throughout years without exhibiting any of the usual symptoms of inflammation like pain or swelling. The initial summoning of white blood cells (inflammatory infiltrate) into the bronchial walls and the interalveolar septum that occurred with the initiation of the smoking history was, for all intents and purposes, the beginning of the chronic inflammatory process. By continuing to constantly irritate the cells lining the respiratory tract with cigarette smoke over the years, the ongoing recruitment of white blood cells was maintained, furthering the process of chronic inflammation. Recurring respiratory infections throughout the years, although acute episodes in their own right, also contributed to perpetuating the presence of white blood cells in the respiratory tract, aiding in the ultimate chronicity of the situation. White blood cells also self–perpetuated their existence by means of molecular messengers. Activated lymphocytes, for example, which are found in the infiltrate of the subepithelial tissue of the bronchial wall, release cytokines (messenger molecules) that in turn stimulate macrophages. Stimulated macrophages in turn release different cytokines that activate more lymphocytes. Leukotrienes (other messenger molecules introduced earlier in this chapter), which are part of the family of eicosanoid molecules that are produced through the arachidonic acid pathway in leukocytes, macrophages, and epithelial cells, are not only chemotactic for (attracts) white blood cells, which ultimately results in the perpetuation of the inflammatory response, but they are also potent initiators of bronchoconstriction. Much more will be said of the arachidonic acid pathway and leukotrienes in chapter 3 as this is one particular area where the nutritional and natural health approaches to reducing inflammation are quite effective and simple to employ.

The continuous presence of white blood cells in the bronchial walls — i.e., the inflammatory cell infiltration that characterizes chronic inflammation — eventually creates a myriad of problems to include edema and peribronchial (area around the bronchi and bronchioles) fibrosis. Tissue necrosis can also occur as a result of chronic inflammation. Whether or not chronic inflammation is causally related to the hypertrophy or hyperplasia that is seen in the submucosal mucous-secreting glands or the mucous-secreting goblet cells is not clear. Hypertrophy and hyperplasia are usually brought about through excessive hormonal stimulation of cells, or through increased functional demands placed on cells. It is also not clear how chronic inflammation is related, if at all, to the atypical metaplasia and dysplasia of the respiratory epithelium that is often seen in patients diagnosed with chronic bronchitis. What is clear, though, is that patients who have atypical metaplasia or dysplasia of the cells in their respiratory tract are at higher risk for developing lung cancer.

This description of chronic inflammation and some of its processes, albeit accurate, is only an overview of an otherwise complex and multifaceted series of events involving many cells and many different types of molecules. It is sufficient, though, to illustrate why, as a result of many years of smoking and recurrent respiratory infections, there is chronic inflammation occurring in the respiratory tract that is a significant component of the overall picture of chronic bronchitis. A comprehensive understanding of the mechanism of chronic inflammation still eludes us; much research must be continued in this area so as to increase our knowledge and provide new methods of treatment. As we close the discussion of emphysema and chronic bronchitis, table 5 compares and contrasts the two conditions according to some of their major features.

Table 5

**Comparison Between Emphysema and Chronic Bronchitis
According to Their Major Features**

Feature	Type A COPD Predominant Emphysema	Type B COPD Predominant Chronic Bronchitis
Location	acinus	bronchi & bronchioles
Major cause	tobacco smoke	tobacco smoke, inhaled irritants
Clinical changes	enlargement of airspaces, alveolar wall destruction	hyperplasia & hypertrophy of mucous glands in respiratory tract
Major symptoms	dyspnea	cough with sputum
Dyspnea	severe, onset is early	mild, onset is late
Cough/sputum	late with slight sputum	early with copious sputum
Elastic recoil	greatly reduced	normal
Airway resistance	normal, slightly increased	increased
Infection	occasional	common
Lung volume	decreased FEV_1 increased TLC & RV	decreased FEV_1 normal TLC, slight RV increase
Body appearance	thin, asthenic, barrel chested, "pink puffer"	adequately nourished, strong, "blue bloater"
Cyanosis	rare	common

Bronchiectasis

Bronchiectasis is characterized by the irreversible dilation and distortion of the bronchi and bronchioles. These airways are abnormally dilated with variable amounts of mucus and inflammation. Normal structural components of the bronchial wall are destroyed and oftentimes replaced by fibrous connective tissue. The exact cause of bronchiectasis is not clearly understood, but it is believed to be a consequence of the manifestation of a cycle between infections, often pneumonia, and inflammation. Recurrent, and thus chronic respiratory infections leads to chronic inflammatory changes that weaken the bronchial walls such that they become dilated and distorted. Mucus and pus accumulate in these dilated areas, which then contributes to the perpetuation of infection. These recurring infections continue to cause even further damage to the lungs, establishing a vicious cycle that becomes increasingly difficult to manage. Bronchiectasis is accompanied by a chronic, loose, productive cough containing significant amounts of foul-smelling sputum.

Although the cause of bronchiectasis is not directly related to cigarette smoking, varying degrees of bronchiectasis are often seen in conjunction with emphysema or chronic bronchitis because of its relationship to chronic infection. The recurrent infections that are characteristic of chronic bronchitis can contribute to exacerbating an already existent condition of bronchiectasis. The main issue therefore in the management of bronchiectasis, as with chronic bronchitis, is to reduce inflammation as much as possible. By reducing inflammation, less mucus will be produced, and with less mucus there will be less propensity for infection. Reduced mucus will also result in a less obstructed airway that will enable easier breathing.

Final remarks

As seen from this chapter, COPD involves pathological changes to the respiratory system that are complex and often overlapping. Insofar as the definition of chronic bronchitis is a clinical definition, the definition of emphysema is anatomical. This means that a diagnosis of chronic bronchitis can be made confidently in a living patient, whereas a definitive diagnosis of emphysema can only be made through an autopsy. Although the medical history, physical examination, various tests, and radiographic studies can indicate with a high degree of probability the presence of emphysema, the amount of emphysematous damage will always remain uncertain. Fortunately, though, knowledge of the precise type of emphysema, or the amount of damage, is not necessary in order to proceed with treatment. Because there are usually elements of both diseases present to varying degrees in any given patient, treatment methodologies are aimed at addressing the symptoms of both emphysema and chronic bronchitis, since both conditions essentially manifest the same problems.

Beginning with the next chapter, this book will make known the steps that can be taken through nutrition and natural/alternative medicine that aim to not only address symptoms, but also to help reduce inflammation and heal tissue, restore biochemical balance, and correct problems at a fundamental level. There is no method yet that can adequately restore the interalveolar septa or alveoli that have been destroyed in emphysema. There is also no means by which to restore the bronchial walls that have become permanently dilated in bronchiectasis. There are, however, many ways available through nutritional and natural medicine to reduce any further destruction, and to strengthen the remaining lung tissue that has not yet been damaged. Control of mucus production and prevention of infection are other big concerns with COPD patients. These are areas that nutritional and natural medicine are quite capable of addressing as part of an overall therapeutic approach whose aim is to build health and lessen the exacerbations that are often seen in COPD.

Chapter 3

Dietary and Nutritional Therapeutics

Introduction

Emphysema and COPD are very challenging illnesses to manage. If, however, you learn to modify your diet and apply the methods and principles of nutritional medicine, you will find that not only can the issues of your COPD improve, but you will also find your general health status improving as well. Nutrition is the cornerstone of health. Period.

The word *diet* as it is used in this chapter does not carry the same meaning as it does when it is used generically to describe, for example, a diet to lose weight. You are not "going on a diet" for COPD. What is implied by the use of the word *diet* as it pertains to COPD is a complete and permanent change in the way in which you eat for the rest of your life. Permanently changing the way in which you eat may prove to be one of the most difficult things you will ever do; however, as you begin to see the difference it makes in the way you feel, and how it can significantly help to lessen the severity of your COPD symptoms, you will come to appreciate your dietary changes as a welcome sacrifice.

It is unfortunate that even today in 2005, most conventional medical schools still only teach a very limited amount of nutrition, and the nutrition that is taught in those medical schools is not usually therapeutic nutrition. This is one of the reasons why most medical doctors are limited in their means to address your health issues from a nutritional standpoint. Doctors of today are indeed highly educated and very well trained, but remember that perspective is everything. The education of a conventional physician, for example, involves coursework in biochemistry, but rarely does it ever involve investigating the nutritional subtleties that very often have significant influence over the regulation of a biochemical pathway. Allopathic (conventional) medical students are taught to use drugs to combat disease, but are rarely, if ever, taught how to use nutrients or dietary protocols to overcome disease. There are obviously times when pharmaceutical intervention is necessary in the treatment of disease, but in the last fifty years since Dr. Abram Hoffer, M.D., Ph.D., and two-time Nobel laureate Dr. Linus Pauling, Ph.D. began the research that laid the groundwork for elucidating the role of nutrition in human health and disease, we have accumulated an overwhelming abundance of scientific evidence that indisputably concludes that the health and wellness of individuals is directly related to, and significantly influenced by, their nutritional status.

Although this book is not intended to address medical education or the state of healthcare delivery in this country, I feel obliged to let you know why most conventional doctors do not have a background in nutritional or natural medicine. Our system of medicine in this country is focused on *disease management* rather than *health promotion*. It is a pharmaceutically driven system. I have no problem with pharmaceutical drugs being used when they are used rationally, meaning that they should only be used when absolutely needed, and always with caution as to their side effects. But this is not how medicine is typically practiced in this country. We have developed assembly-line medicine where you are processed through the system, see a doctor for ten minutes, get your prescription, and then you're on your way. Somewhere along the way, and for reasons too manifold and complex to be within the scope of this book, the conventional system lost some of its perspective on being an institution whose charge was to genuinely care for the well-being of people, and instead it became a less sensitive, automated, highly bureaucratic institution that found itself under the control of business entities that oftentimes put cost containment, profit, and self-satisfaction ahead of the health and welfare of human beings.

The current healthcare system of today has left countless numbers of individuals dissatisfied with the care they have received. This is why so many people are turning to holistic medical doctors, naturopaths and other types of alternative practitioners for their healthcare needs. I have known many fine, well-intentioned M.D.'s whose hearts and minds were in the right place, that have become completely disgusted with the way the system of medical practice has evolved in this country over the last several decades. They all share the same sorrow over being dictated to by the insurance companies and the drug corporations as to how they must practice medicine today.

But realize, and this is the crux of this message, that even the "open-minded" medical doctors of today, despite being well-intended and at odds with the bureaucrats that dictate medical practice, unless they have received additional training, are still for the most part not versed in the methods of nutritional medicine because they were never taught it in medical school. These doctors, however, because of their caring dispositions and inclinations toward being open-minded, are more likely to work with you in learning about nutritional medicine because of their motivation to help you. Any doctor whose care you are under for the treatment of COPD should be most willing to work with you to implement the methods and strategies contained in this book. If you find yourself in the predicament where your physician or pulmonologist is not willing to explore the options and methods within this book, I would suggest finding another physician who is willing to support you in your choice to utilize nutritional and natural health means to rebuild your health. Appendix 3 at the end of this book provides a generous list of organizations that will be able to help you find a physician or other natural health practitioner that has had the appropriate training in nutritional and natural medicine that can work with you in implementing the strategies contained in this book.

As much as the predicament of the modern healthcare system grieves me, I honestly do not have a short answer on how to solve the complex and very messy problems that plague the healthcare system of today. What I did come to realize, though, is that through writing I could make an impact that would make a difference in people's lives. I realized that if I chose a career that focused predominantly on researching and writing about the natural and alternative therapeutic approaches to health, I could reach infinitely more people with the useful information they need to improve their health. I thought one day back when I was in medical school that even if I saw forty patients a day for the rest of my working life, I would never be able to see enough people to even make a dent in the number of people who have emphysema or COPD. It then came as a surprise to me to find out that there was no book in existence that addressed this disease from the perspective of natural or alternative medicine. This is one of the main reasons that drove me to writing this book; I knew that unless someone wrote specifically about the therapeutic approaches to COPD through nutrition and natural medicine, you would probably never get this information in a single source. I knew you would probably never get this information from your physician, yet I also knew from experience that because it was so useful, it was information that was necessary for you and your physician to have.

In the twelve years since I began researching the natural and alternative therapeutic approaches to emphysema and COPD, I have amassed a considerable amount of information. My college, medical school, and naturopathy school background, along with my experience, has enabled me to distill all that I have researched such that I will not only be writing about what is capable of being effective and practical, but I will also explain why I believe the methods I present are legitimate. Let us now begin our discussion of therapeutic approaches to COPD as it pertains to diet and nutrition.

The role of nutrition

As research in nutritional biochemistry continues to unfold new information regarding the role of nutrients in human metabolism, we not only acquire a better understanding of the relationship between nutrition and health, but we also discover how nutritional intervention can be useful in the eradication of illness. We all know that we are supposed to "eat right" in order to be healthy, but most people have probably never really been taught what it means to have a truly nutritional diet. The consequences of what we believe to be an acceptable diet are all around us. Heart disease, morbid obesity, cancer, and type II diabetes are just some of the health issues that can be directly related to the compromised nutritional status that results from the modern American diet. The concept of nutrition that you may be most familiar with that consists of the four food groups, the food pyramid, and the recommended daily allowance for nutrients is far from correct. Yes, there are some generalizations that can be made regarding nutritional requirements, and even though the recommended daily allowance for nutrients may prevent some of the more severe deficiency diseases, the prevailing conventional concept of what constitutes adequate nutrition is a long way off from what is really needed in order to be building optimal health. Science is now showing us that the nutritional requirements for any one particular individual are unique and specific to that individual. What we are really beginning to understand is the concept of biochemical individuality where the amounts of nutrients that individuals need to maintain optimal health vary according to their own unique biochemical needs. The emerging branch of medicine known as orthomolecular medicine is the field of medicine that uses a wide range of diagnostic tests to access a person's individual nutritional status. Orthomolecular physicians, through a variety of tests, are able to assess the specific nutritional needs for any one particular individual. These tests are also able to reveal any nutritional deficiencies that, if not corrected, can lead to future health problems.

While it is true that many health problems are the result of certain nutritional deficiencies, this is not the case with emphysema or COPD. Even emphysema cases that are attributed to an alpha 1 AT deficiency are not considered to be due to a nutritional deficiency as this is not an issue where the body is deficient in a nutrient, but rather it is a deficiency due to the improper expression of a protein because of a genetic mutation. On the other hand, though, as a result of all your years of smoking and having what would be considered a less than nutritionally sound diet, you have acquired additional nutritional needs that need to be met in order to start turning your health around. Your smoking and less-than-optimal diet have put stress on more than just your lungs. As the body's major detoxifying organ, your liver has been subjected to undue stress due to all the toxicity it has been subjected to from cigarettes and a nutritionally poor diet. The consequences of your COPD have also put increased stress on your kidneys and your heart. And furthermore, if your intestines are not working optimally, you will have problems with the absorption of nutrients that will provoke additional problems.

Emphysema or COPD has taken its toll on all of you, not just your lungs. Now the main focus of this book is going to be addressing the issues directly related to your respiratory system, but I cannot emphasize enough that in order for you to comprehensively turn your health around, you need to be working with either a naturopath, or a holistic medical doctor, who understands the interrelationships of the body's systems such that he or she can orchestrate a truly holistic program of nutritional care that will address the entirety of your body's needs. In so doing, not only will you curb your immediate COPD symptoms, but you will also be working to correct any other problems you may have so as to ultimately improve your overall health.

The fact that you have significant problems with your respiratory system due to your COPD is quite obvious because of all the symptoms you manifest on a daily basis. Whether it is shortness of breath, constant coughing of mucus, or recurrent respiratory infections, these are all signs of COPD that let you know your respiratory system is in trouble. But do not be deceived into thinking that just because you do not experience the symptoms of liver problems, or because you haven't had heart trouble, this means that these organs are all okay. They are not necessarily okay. If you have any degree of emphysema or COPD, you definitely need to address the nutritional needs of your liver. Depending on the severity of your COPD, you may have already begun to experience heart trouble. Cor pulmonale (an abnormal enlargement of the right ventricle of the heart due to hypertension of the pulmonary circulation) is commonly seen with chronic bronchitis, and it is also seen at the end stages of emphysema.

Hopefully, you are beginning to see that despite being diagnosed with emphysema or COPD, in order to get your health turned around, you are going to have to address a lot more than just your respiratory system. This is why I say again that it is so important for you to work with a healthcare provider who is capable of assessing and understanding the entirety of your specific nutritional requirements. If you begin now to identify the other areas of weakness in your body besides your lungs, you can utilize nutritional medicine to make the necessary corrections now and hopefully avert the need for more invasive or aggressive intervention later. You have enough on your plate already in dealing with your everyday respiratory struggles, so minimize or eliminate any future problems that your COPD has instigated with other parts of your body by initiating the appropriate nutritional protocols today.

Through a program of proper nutritional intervention, you will not only be addressing the symptoms of your COPD, but you will also be aiding your body in the restoration of your overall health. This is accomplished because of the synergistic way in which nutritional and dietary protocols act upon your body. Even though some of the dietary and nutritional methods that will be introduced in this chapter are aimed at helping to reduce specific symptoms, because of the synergistic way in which these methods act upon your body, they bring about their results in a manner that is edifying to your whole body. This is quite different from the way pharmaceutical drugs act. This is most evidenced by the fact that pharmaceutical drugs have side effects, often very deleterious side effects, whereas dietary and nutritional methods usually do not. This is one of the major benefits of natural medicine.

It is necessary that you see the restoration of your health as a project that you have undertaken where you are the one in the driver's seat. It is a project that needs to be actively maintained and will require your continuous, attentive involvement. This is the only way that nutritional and natural medicine can effectively work. You are going to learn to listen to, and understand, your body in a way that you probably never imagined before. There is no quick fix in natural medicine. Because there are so many nuances related to your condition, and so much variety amongst the protocols that can be used to bring about restoration of your health, you will play an integral role in reading your own body in determining what specific protocols are working for you. This book will lay the groundwork for the therapeutic choices that are available, and your doctor will assist and guide you as you navigate your way through the choices, but ultimately you are the one that will steer yourself on the road to health.

The following list indicates the therapeutic goals most COPD patients would like to be able to accomplish. The nutritional methods available to address these issues are abundant. As you begin to make changes in the way you eat, and begin to introduce nutritional supplements and herbs into your diet, as well as all the other natural and alternative methods that you will eventually employ as part of your process to regain your health, keep these goals in mind and monitor your progress as you begin to see achievements in the areas that matter to you the most.

Therapeutic goals (not necessarily in order of priority):

- Repair and healing of damaged tissue to the extent that is scientifically possible
- Increased breathing capacity with greater airflow through the airways
- Management and control of mucus production
- Management and control of inflammation
- Prevention of infection and strengthening of immunity
- Increased vitality
- Increased ability to exercise and exert energy
- Decreased dependency on pharmaceutical drugs as much as possible
- Improvement of overall health status

Let us now begin to explore the specifics of what can be done from a nutritional and dietary perspective to curb the symptoms of COPD and start turning your health around.

The medicinal use of food for COPD

This is the section where the rubber meets the road. Beginning in this section and for the remainder of the book, you are going to discover the choices available to address both the symptoms of your COPD and the improvement of your overall health. Of all the options that you will discover in this book, the dietary considerations you are about to read may in all likelihood be the most difficult for you to tackle. Changing the way you eat is much more difficult than taking supplements or herbs, but hear me clearly when I say that making the necessary changes to your diet is the single most important thing you can do for your condition, and furthermore, if you don't change your diet, all the other steps you take will for the most part be much less effective in bringing about any significant change in your condition. If you need to take your time in adjusting to this new way of eating, just remember that the stricter you are with yourself in adhering to the dietary strategies, the better your results will be. If you are faithful to consistently comply with the guidelines outlined — and consistent compliance means daily compliance for the rest of your life — you will find your dilemma with COPD much easier to manage.

<u>Foods to Avoid</u>

The major issues that will be addressed through the avoidance of certain foods are reducing inflammation and mucus production, and relieving bronchoconstriction. Reducing mucus and inflammation will result in an increase in breathing capacity as well as reducing your susceptibility to infection. These are all central issues associated with COPD that can be effectively addressed with consistent compliance to the following dietary restrictions.

Animal foods (red meat, liver, brain, chicken skin, shellfish, mollusks, egg yolks, and all dairy products, especially milk, cheese, and butterfat): The elimination of these animal foods from the diet plays a significant role in reducing both mucus and inflammation. Red meat and dairy products are known mucus-forming foods, and by eliminating them from your diet you will not only reduce the mucus production in your lungs, but mucus formation will also be reduced in your intestines, sinuses, and your nasal cavity as well. Perhaps the most striking feature, though, of eliminating animal foods from your diet is that it will have a similar anti–inflammatory effect on your body as some of the steroid drugs you may be familiar with, yet without the side effects of these drugs that you are probably all too familiar with. Allow me to explain this. Back in chapter 2 in the section headed "chronic bronchitis — inflammation," messenger molecules involved in the inflammatory process known as leukotrienes and cytokines were introduced. A messenger molecule is a compound that essentially enables one cell to communicate with another cell. There are a variety of ways in which cells can communicate with one another throughout the body. Some cells produce messenger molecules that are released into the bloodstream where they travel some distance before reaching their target cells. Other cells produce messengers that do not enter systemic circulation, but rather they exert their action locally amongst the cells in their immediate area. One particular group of these local acting messengers, collectively known as the eicosanoids, consists of messenger molecules known as leukotrienes, prostaglandins, prostacyclins, and thromboxanes. As molecular messengers, the eicosanoid molecules play a significant role in blood coagulation, vasodilation, vasoconstriction, bronchoconstriction, and regulation of the inflammatory response.

As far as the inflammation that occurs with COPD is concerned, the main pro–inflammatory eicosanoid that contributes to perpetuating inflammation in the walls of the bronchi and bronchioles is LTB_4 (leukotriene B_4). LTB_4 causes increased chemotaxis of leukocytes into the bronchial wall. Essentially this means that LTB_4, through its messaging action, recruits white blood cells into the bronchial wall, and this contributes to the perpetuation of the inflammatory condition of the bronchial wall. There are other leukotrienes (LTC_4, LTD_4, and LTE_4) that are also problematic for individuals with COPD as these leukotrienes cause bronchoconstriction by inducing the contraction of smooth muscle in the lungs.

The source of the significant 4-series leukotrienes (LTB_4, LTC_4, LTD_4, and LTE_4) is the precursor molecule known as arachidonic acid. Arachidonic acid, which resides in the cell membrane, is obtained in two ways. The vast majority of the body's arachidonic acid supply is obtained through the diet, and the dietary sources of arachidonic acid are the animal foods listed in boldface at the beginning of this section. Arachidonic acid is also formed as a result of a biochemical pathway where linoleic acid (an omega–6 essential fatty acid found in the cell membrane) is converted into arachidonic acid. Arachidonic acid is released from the cell membrane and enters into the cytoplasm through the action of the enzyme phospholipase A_2. Figure 7 illustrates a simplification of the biochemical pathway of linoleic acid being converted into arachidonic acid, which then gets converted into the leukotrienes (LTB_4, LTC_4, LTD_4, and LTE_4).

Figure 7   **Generalized summary of the portion of the arachidonic acid pathway leading to 4 series leukotriene formation.**

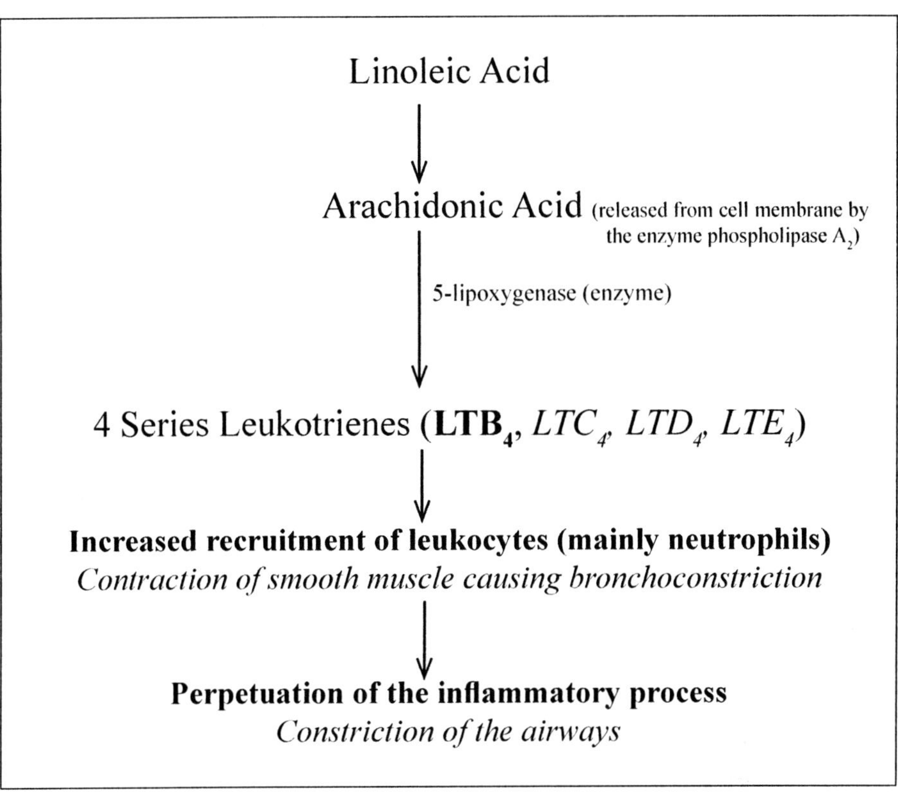

If you are a COPD patient, you are more than likely all too familiar with the steroidal anti–inflammatory drug Prednisone. It has probably been prescribed for you at times when your inflammation was particularly severe. Prednisone in my opinion should only be used as a very last resort because of its dangerous and damaging side effects. Prednisone effectively reduces inflammation by inhibiting phospholipase A_2 (see figure 7). When phospholipase A_2 is inhibited, arachidonic acid cannot be released from the cell membrane, and without the release of arachidonic acid the pro–inflammatory eicosanoids cannot be produced. This is a powerful way to reduce inflammation, but at what price? Prednisone is known to commonly cause the following side effects:

1)   Sodium retention — this will raise your blood pressure as well as increase the viscosity of your mucus secretions
2)   Increased fat deposits
3)   Increased acid in your stomach
4)   Increased sweating, especially at night
5)   Hyperglycemia (elevated blood sugar levels)
6)   Photosensitivity (increased sensitivity to the sun)
7)   Thrush (Candida) growth in the mouth
8)   Bone, muscle, and eye problems
9)   Acne on the face, back, and chest
10)   Decreased ability to fight infection
11)   Delayed wound healing
12)   Vulnerability to depression
13)   Nausea, vomiting, and peptic ulcers
14)   Suppression of the adrenal gland
15)   Cataracts and increased intraocular pressure

Is all this worth it, when you can effectively reduce inflammation and lessen bronchoconstriction by just not eating the animal foods listed in this section? If you stop eating red meat, liver, brain, shellfish, mollusks, and dairy products, you will have effectively eliminated the dietary sources of arachidonic acid. Your body will still be able to manufacture arachidonic acid from linoleic acid on an as-needed basis, but in terms of the overall picture, by eliminating your dietary intake of these animal foods, which are the body's main source of arachidonic acid, you will produce considerably less leukotriene B_4, and as a result you will reduce the inflammatory response that is occurring in your bronchial walls. Furthermore, as it pertains to your body making arachidonic acid from linoleic acid, the last enzyme in the sequence of steps that converts linoleic acid to arachidonic acid is known as $\Delta 5$ desaturase. $\Delta 5$ desaturase prefers omega–3 fatty acids, which means that if you increase your intake of omega–3 rich foods such as cold–water fish and flax seed, when it comes to your body making arachidonic acid from linoleic acid, since $\Delta 5$ desaturase prefers omega–3 fatty acids, it will opt to facilitate the conversion of these omega–3 fatty acids into eicosapentaenoic acid (EPA) rather than facilitating the conversion of linoleic acid into arachidonic acid. This means that you will end up producing more of the favorable 3 series prostaglandins rather than the pro–inflammatory and bronchoconstricting 4 series leukotrienes and pro–inflammatory 2 series prostaglandins. With less inflammation and bronchoconstriction occurring in your bronchial walls, your airway will become less obstructed, mucus production will be lessened, and you will ultimately be able to breathe easier. Unless you are an infant who is in need of arachidonic acid for brain development, or you are a nursing mother providing an infant with arachidonic acid through your breast milk, there will be no negative consequences from eliminating these animal foods from your diet.

White flour products (white bread, pasta, and many cereals): The issue here again is mucus. White flour products, because of the chemical bleaching they undergo in processing, are bad food choices to begin with, but because wheat in general is mucus forming due to the gluten it contains, it is an even worse choice for a COPD patient. It is extremely important that you read labels very carefully as there are many other food products that contain wheat flour as an additive or filler. Millers also oftentimes mix wheat flour with other nonwheat flours such as oats. Safe alternatives to these restrictions that are good choices for you are nuts, seeds, nonwheat whole grains, and flour products that are made from amaranth, kamut, corn, brown rice, quinoa, and spelt. Pasta made from the flour derived from either brown rice, kamut, quinoa, or spelt are all excellent alternatives to regular white flour pasta made from semolina.

Salt: Increased sodium (salt) concentration in your blood results in water being drawn from the tissues into the blood to lower the concentration of salt. This not only raises blood pressure, but in your case, it also results in a lessening of the amount of water in the tissue of your bronchi and bronchioles. This causes the mucus in your respiratory tract to become thicker and more viscous. Excessive salt also promotes the raising of histamine levels, which further provokes the inflammatory process.

Fried and greasy foods: Avoid all fried and greasy foods as these foods are not only bad for you for a myriad of other reasons, but they too are mucus forming and contribute to the inflammation in your bronchial wall.

Processed foods, junk foods, and refined sugar: Processed foods and junk foods (the majority of what you find in a box or can in your typical grocery store) are very detrimental to you as a COPD patient. Processed foods and junk foods are full of additives and artificial ingredients, all of which are toxic to your body and contribute to inflammation, formation of mucus, and the weakening of your immune system. You need to read labels very carefully and avoid all processed foods and refined sugar. Junk food and sweets will aggravate your condition considerably if you are not careful. Refined sugar, candy, soda pop, and snack foods, although they are tasty and desirable, should be avoided as much as possible by someone with COPD. Avoid also all the artificial sweeteners that are available today. Use honey sparingly as a sweetener when necessary.

Caffeine and alcohol: Avoid coffee, black tea, and alcohol in any form as these are all dehydrating and very deleterious to your system. Caffeine, however, because of its effectiveness as a bronchodilator, can be used to induce relaxation of the bronchial passages and facilitate easier breathing. The use of caffeine for this purpose should be limited to only when absolutely necessary to help breathing in a situation of acute dyspnea where nothing else is available to help you.

Gas-forming foods: Depending upon your situation, you may need to avoid cabbage and legumes. Legumes are peas, lentils, peanuts, beans, and other plant foods that are found in pods. These foods tend to be gas–forming and may cause abdominal distention that can make breathing more difficult.

<u>Foods You Should Be Eating Regularly</u>

Raw foods: Ideally, in your situation as an emphysema or COPD patient, your diet should consist of at least 50 percent raw organic food. If you have severe inflammation associated with chronic bronchitis, I would recommend increasing this percentage to 75 percent. The concept of eating a raw foods diet will in all likelihood seem very strange to you at first, but, in all honesty, this will be one of the smartest moves you can make insofar as your condition is concerned. It is not by accident that people who subscribe to a predominantly raw foods diet are some of the healthiest people on the planet. A raw foods diet is one of the best possible sources of proper nutrition (including protein) available. Making raw foods a substantial part of your diet is going to enable your body to detoxify properly and build immunity, significantly reduce inflammation and mucus formation, thereby allowing you to breathe easier, help you to regain energy and strength, and provide for you a new level of vitality and mental acuity. You will have to determine, depending upon your circumstances, the extent to which you are willing or able to adopt this style of eating. I highly recommend, if it is at all possible, to give this area a serious effort, as the health benefits and the degree of resolve it will bring to your condition are considerable.

A raw foods diet (raw–vegan) means eating foods (plant foods) in their natural, uncooked state. This style of eating is not something you just jump into. You will need guidance to help you learn how to eat this way. There are many sources of information and books on how to successfully incorporate this way of eating into your life. There are three great books that I would recommend. The first book, *12 Steps to Raw Foods: How to End Your Addiction to Cooked Food,* by Victoria Boutenko, is an excellent place to start if you have never experienced eating a raw foods diet before. Two other excellent books packed with recipes and tons of information on eating raw foods are the following: *The Complete Book of Raw Food: Healthy, Delicious Vegetarian Cuisine Made with Living Foods,* by Julie Rodwell, and *Living Cuisine: The Art and Spirit of Raw Foods,* by Renee Loux Underkoffler. The staff at your local farmer's market or organic/whole foods grocery store will also be a great source of information. There are recipes available that enable you to have a raw food version of whatever you may have thought you were craving from your old style of eating. Raw food preparation and variety has actually reached the level of being as much of an art form as conventional cuisine. Salads, fresh vegetables, avocados, bananas, nut-milk, tomatoes, humus, wheat grass juice, raisins, seaweed, fresh fruits of all types, pumpkin and sunflower seeds, fresh-squeezed citrus juices, vegetable juices, almonds, sprouts, dried apricots, berries — these are but a few of the hundreds and hundreds of food choices you will have within the world of raw foods eating. Be sure, though, that within this vast variety of choices you always include dark green leafy and purple/red varieties of vegetables, beets, radishes, red onions, chives, blue, purple, and dark red berries, pineapples, and papayas. Be mindful that sweet fruits can tend to be mucus forming, so limit yourself in the amount of sweet fruit you consume. Sweet fruits are fruits like dates, bananas, dried fruit, figs, and persimmon. Also remember that cold–pressed olive oil, flaxseed oil, and hempseed oil are the only types of oils you want to be using in any of your preparations.

Organic poultry, cold–water fish, dairy substitutes, vegetable-based soups, and nonwheat flour products: Skinless organic chicken or turkey, as well as cold–water fish such as salmon, albacore tuna, rainbow trout, herring, mackerel, whiting, sardines, and pilchards are all acceptable food choices for sources of protein. These fishes are also excellent sources of the omega–3 essential fatty acids EPA and DHA, both of which have well-established anti–inflammatory properties. EPA and DHA both competitively inhibit the conversion of arachidonic acid to leukotriene B_4, as well as inhibiting the conversion of arachidonic acid to the pro–inflammatory 2 series prostaglandins. Other excellent sources of protein are tofu and most of the different varieties of beans. Soymilk, rice milk, almond milk, and coconut milk are great choices to substitute for regular milk. Even animal-derived organic milk is still not a good choice for you because it will contain pro-inflammatory arachidonic acid, although goat's milk is less inflammatory than cow's milk. Remember to maintain adequate calcium intake in light of your abstinence from dairy products. Excellent sources of dietary calcium are dark green leafy vegetables, asparagus, broccoli, kale, soybeans, tofu, and watercress. You may even consider taking supplemental calcium if needed. As you make food choices for yourself, remember to orchestrate your diet within the context of a predominantly raw foods diet so as to gain the maximum therapeutic benefit for your COPD. Black bean soup (made with vegetable-based stock) prepared with onions and garlic is particularly useful as an anti–inflammatory. Non–white flour products that are made from amaranth, kamut, corn flour, brown rice, quinoa, and spelt will provide alternatives for breads, muffins, and pasta that you will be able to enjoy without causing mucus formation or aggravating your condition.

Hot and spicy foods: To the extent that your palate can tolerate, foods such as onions, garlic, various types of chilis, mustard, and horseradish will all benefit your condition. These foods are stimulating to your immune system and help provide nourishment to your respiratory system. Furthermore, garlic and onions both contain quercetin, a flavonoid compound that research has shown to inhibit lipoxygenase (see figure 7). Inhibition of lipoxygenase means that the production of 4 series leukotrienes will be lessened, which will result in less bronchoconstriction and chemotaxis of leukocytes, and a consequent reduction in inflammation. Research also indicates that quercetin can also inhibit pro–inflammatory 2 series prostaglandins. Now to the extent that you can eliminate your dietary sources of arachidonic acid, thereby lessening the formation of 4 series leukotrienes and the inflammation and bronchoconstriction they cause, recall that your body can still make arachidonic acid from linoleic acid. The quercetin contained in garlic and onions, however, will aid in preventing the arachidonic acid that is formed this way from being converted into 4 series leukotrienes by inhibiting 5–lipoxygenase, the enzyme that is necessary to ultimately convert arachidonic acid into 4 series leukotrienes. Through elimination of the animal foods listed earlier in this chapter, increasing your intake of omega–3 rich foods, and increasing your dietary intake of garlic and onions, you will very effectively inhibit the formation of pro–inflammatory 2 series prostaglandins and 4 series leukotrienes. You will reduce bronchoconstriction, inflammation and the production of mucus, which will enable you to breathe easier and lower your susceptibility to infection. Taking supplemental quercetin will further enhance the inhibition of 4 series leukotrienes and the pro–inflammatory 2 series prostaglandins. This will be discussed in more detail in chapter 4. Table 6 provides a comprehensive summary of foods that are to be avoided, as well as the foods that are either beneficial or acceptable in the diet of an individual with COPD.

Table 6

<table>
<tr><td colspan="2" align="center">Diet and Food Summary</td></tr>
<tr><td align="center">Avoid</td><td align="center">Good choices</td></tr>
<tr><td valign="top">

Animal foods: red meat, liver, brain chicken skin, shellfish, mollusks, & egg yolks
Dairy products: especially milk, cheese, butterfat, & margarine
White flour products: bread, pasta, cereals derived from white flour, rye, oats, barley, & whole wheat
Salt
Processed foods & junk foods
Refined sugar: candy, snack foods, soda pop, & artificial sweeteners
Fried & greasy foods
Caffeine & alcohol
Allergenic foods

</td><td valign="top">

Raw foods: all fresh organic fruits & vegetables, nuts, seeds, & non–wheat whole grains
Cold–pressed olive oil
Hot & spicy foods: onions, garlic, chilis, mustard, & horseradish
Skinless organic poultry
Cold–water fish: salmon, albacore tuna, rainbow trout, herring, whiting, mackerel, sardines, & pilchards
Tofu
Soy, rice, coconut, or almond milk
Nonwheat flour products: corn flour, brown rice flour, amaranth, kamut, quinoa, & spelt
Honey: sparingly as a sweetener

</td></tr>
</table>

Proper food combining

To ensure proper digestion and to help reduce mucus formation and inflammation, it is essential to combine foods appropriately. The following guidelines will show you how to combine food properly when eating so as to streamline digestion, reduce mucus formation, and energize and strengthen your body.

1. Do not eat proteins and starches together. Proteins and starches eaten together tend to spoil in the stomach, cause indigestion and fatigue, and promote weight gain.

2. Do not eat proteins with fats or oils.

3. Eat proteins as a main course with vegetables and a salad.

4. Eat starches as a main course with vegetables and a salad.

5. Always eat fruit by itself on an empty stomach. Allow a half-hour to pass after eating fruit before eating other foods. Melon should be eaten either alone or before other fruits. Sweet fruits should be eaten after other fruits.

6. You may eat nuts with acid fruits.

7. Avocados combine well with all foods except proteins and melons.

8. Tomatoes may be combined with nonstarchy vegetables and protein.

The chart on the following page is a guide to proper food combining. You may combine together the foods that are directly connected by an arrow. You may only combine two boxes at a time. Melon has no arrows connecting it to anything else as it should always be eaten alone.

Proper food–combining for efficient digestion and minimization of inflammation and mucus

Foods that are *directly* connected by an arrow may be eaten together at the same meal

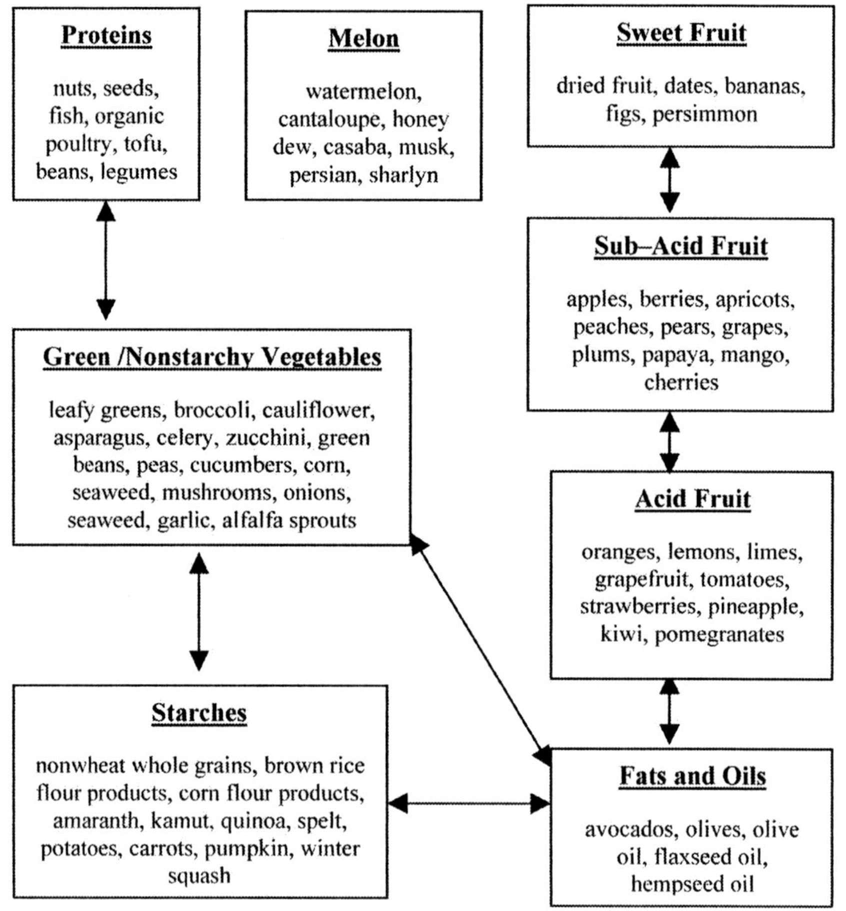

Juicing and detoxification

Juicing raw vegetables and fruits is particularly beneficial to persons with COPD. Fresh raw juices deliver high-quality, concentrated nutrients to your body that are usually assimilated within thirty minutes. In order to obtain maximum nutritional benefit from juicing, it is important for you to prepare fresh juice yourself rather than buying it from the store. Commercial juice is usually pasteurized, a process that uses heat to destroy microorganisms and prolong the product's shelf life. The heat of the pasteurization process, however, also destroys many of the nutrients in the juice. Even some of the highest-quality commercial juice products that utilize "flash pasteurization" still lose valuable nutrients in this process. By using your own juicer, you assure yourself that the juice you prepare is pure, tasty, free of any additives or preservatives, and complete with all the nutritional value that nature intended.

Juicing, in similar fashion to eating raw foods, has demonstrated health benefits that are incalculable. Specifically as it relates to COPD, juicing is excellent as a means to reduce inflammation and mucus, detoxify the body and build immunity so as to increase resistance to infection and increase your vitality, and can significantly aid in the improvement of your overall health status. The fresh juices of the following fruits and vegetables are particularly noteworthy in their usefulness with COPD:

aloe vera   celery   grape   carrot   broccoli   radish   beet root watercress   cucumber   wheatgrass   leafy greens (especially spinach, kale, and dark green vegetables)

Depending upon the severity of your COPD, I would recommend from two to four 8-ounce glasses of fresh juice daily. If your inflammation and mucus are light to moderate, and you are otherwise not experiencing any current exacerbation of your condition, two 8-ounce glasses per day will suffice. If your inflammation and mucus are severe, try drinking four 8-ounce glasses a day until your condition resolves, and then maintain two 8-ounce glasses per day as a daily regimen. Make sure that you always vary the juices from the list and that you rotate through all of them regularly. You may also want to put a small amount of garlic juice into your raw vegetable juice, as the garlic juice will enhance the therapeutic efficacy of the raw vegetable juice.

Once you obtain a juicer if you do not already have one, you will need to find a good source of quality organic produce and begin learning how to prepare produce for juicing. Juicing fresh produce is a fun and easy process to learn, but it does have some particularities that need to be understood, and in order to become well familiarized with the process, I recommend reading any of the following books on juicing: *Juicing for Life* by Julie Calbom, *The Juiceman's Power of Juicing* by Jay Kordich, or *The Juicing Bible* by Pat Crocker. These books are all very well reputed and will give you a tremendous amount of information on all aspects of juicing. I recommend these books, because next to eating raw foods, consuming fresh vegetable juices is one of the most important things that you need to be doing to address your COPD as far as nutritional therapeutics is concerned.

The scope of this chapter has been primarily to make you aware of the food choices you need to be making, or not making, in order to gain the most therapeutic benefit for your COPD. Beyond that scope, however, as it pertains to the areas of raw foods eating and juicing, is information that is important enough to warrant further attention. I have given recommendations for other books to be read in the area of raw foods and juicing as these two areas well deserve to be further explored in detail by every COPD patient. Reading and learning more about eating raw foods and juicing will enable you to maximize their therapeutic benefits. The superior abilities of regular juicing and a raw foods diet to effect significant improvements with COPD, as well as making major contributions to your overall health, cannot be emphasized enough. Through your continued exploration of raw foods and juicing, you will come to develop strategies that work best for the specifics of your case. Once you begin to see the improvements that these strategies make with your COPD, as well as the overall health benefits that these two methods bring to your life, I would hope that you would maintain juicing and eating raw foods as a permanent feature of your overall diet.

Incorporating juicing and eating raw foods into your diet is a prime example of what I was referring to earlier in this chapter in the section on the role of nutrition where I said that you have to see the restoration of your health as a project in which you are in the driver's seat. As far as nutritional therapeutics is concerned, there are areas that are black and white and areas that are gray. Avoiding all the foods covered in the "foods to avoid" section of this chapter is a black-and-white issue. They are simply foods that you should not eat because they will definitely aggravate your condition. Proper food combining is also a black-and-white issue because it has been clearly established that through proper food combining, you will definitely digest your food more efficiently and avoid contributing to the inflammation, mucus formation, and other problems that result from improper digestion. Eating raw foods and juicing, though, are black and white to the extent that these two methods are well established means to help you improve your condition, but they are gray in the sense that you have huge variety in terms of what is available to you in your design of a raw foods diet, or in your selection of juices. This is why I refer to you being in the driver's seat for these two areas. You will have to exercise a higher degree of personal involvement in order to ascertain which choices are working best for you.

Hopefully you see this in a positive light as the process of learning what will work for you is healing in and of itself. I thoroughly realize that oftentimes the predicament of a COPD patient is very difficult, and that you may not want to be belabored with too many choices, as you are primarily concerned with alleviating your physical symptoms as quickly as possible. The dietary protocols laid out in this chapter will help to bring you resolve with your symptomatic issues if you are faithful in your compliance, but remember that healing involves all of you, not just your physical symptoms. If you have COPD as a result of smoking cigarettes, try to understand that from a mental or spiritual perspective, it was because at some point in your past many years ago you allowed your will to be yielded over to an addiction that you knew was going to be very harmful to your health. You remained preoccupied with that pattern of addictive harmful behavior until it got you to where you are now. Insofar as this book is not about addressing the issues of addiction, of which I am no expert, what I want you to take home from this paragraph is that by embracing the new responsibility you have with regard to learning about eating raw foods and juicing, you assume the unique position where you are able to be directly involved in making positive choices for yourself that will ultimately have a beneficial, healthful impact upon your life. This is part of healing. At a deeper level, it's not just that the cigarettes themselves were harmful to you, although they most certainly were; it's the fact that you *chose* to smoke them in the first place. The mental aspect of your decision to start smoking was just as harmful to you as the physical damage that cigarettes have done to your body. Something about you allowed yourself to begin and sustain a behavior that you knew full well to be very dangerous. The aspect of you that enabled you to yield your will and chose to engage in harmful behavior needs to be healed every bit as much as your physical body. By becoming actively involved in making healthy choices for yourself now insofar as your raw foods diet and juicing are concerned, you have an opportunity to reassume control of that part of your will in a positive way, and that will contribute greatly to the healing that is also needed in your mind or your spirit. You will have many more opportunities for involvement as you progress through this book. All the remaining chapters of this book will have areas that are black and white and areas where you will have choice. May you seize every opportunity available to not only help your body but also strengthen your mind or your spirit, through the benefits that are derived by being actively involved in making healthy, positive choices for yourself.

In order for dietary and nutritional therapeutics, as well as nutritional supplementation and herbal medicine for that matter, to have maximal effect on the body, it is necessary for them to be at work in a clean, nontoxic environment. Inadequate digestion, or undigested residue lingering in the bowel, will interfere with the proper absorption and uptake into the blood circulation of the nutrients that you are attempting to assimilate to help with your COPD. It is therefore important to detoxify your digestive system and your bowel in order to ensure that you obtain maximum absorption and effectiveness of the nutritional protocols you are employing. To this end I recommend always ensuring that you have more than adequate amounts of fiber in your diet. Psyllium is one of the best fiber supplements available to ensure regularity of the bowel. Of the many varieties of supplemental fiber to choose from, I personally recommend *Super Colon Cleanse* by Health Plus, Inc. This formula provides a full gram of pysllium husk per serving along with the herbs senna, fennel seed, peppermint, papaya, rose hips, buckthorn bark, barberry root, celery, as well as acidophilus. It would also be beneficial to initiate the cleansing of your bowel by having a colonic irrigation procedure done by a physician. This is essentially a high-tech enema that has to be done in the office, and it is very effective at cleansing the bowel of toxic debris. If this is not possible for you, then as a second choice I would recommend regular enemas on a weekly basis. If you incorporate raw foods eating and juicing into your daily diet, this in and of itself will contribute immensely to the detoxification of not only your digestive system but your entire body as well.

Fasting is also often part of the detoxification process; however, for persons who have emphysema or COPD, I am not going to recommend fasting. Depending upon your condition, it is entirely possible that your body is in too fragile of a state for you to be able to safely fast. If you want to incorporate fasting as part of a detoxification protocol, I would not do so unless it was at the advice of, and under the direct supervision of, your physician.

The last thing I want to discuss regarding detoxification is the role played by your liver in the detoxification process. Your liver is the major detoxifying organ in your body. It is in the liver that the toxins we inhale and ingest are metabolized and broken down so that they may be eliminated. Toxins from the food we eat, the water we drink, and the air we breathe are all metabolized and broken down by the liver. Tobacco smoke, prescription drugs, and nonprescription over-the-counter medicines are all included. Essentially everything you breathe in, or put in your mouth, must be metabolized by your liver. If you are diagnosed with COPD, there is no doubt that you must give your liver some attention. Years of smoking and poor nutritional habits have put significant stress on your liver. It's not to say that your liver is in trouble, it's only that you want to give your liver some additional support in light of the extra work it has to do insofar as your condition is concerned. Cigarettes themselves have caused immense oxidative stress, as it was your liver that had to break down and metabolize several thousand toxic chemicals every time you lighted up a cigarette. In order to support your liver, and help it to operate efficiently, it would be a good idea to supplement with lipotropic factors. Lipotropic formulas are manufactured by most major manufacturers of nutritional supplements. They usually contain choline, methionine, betaine, folic acid, and vitamins B6 and B12. They promote improved liver function and fat metabolism by enhancing the flow of bile and fat to and from the liver. The extract from the seeds of the milk thistle plant, which contains the flavonoid compound silymarin, has impressive research results indicating its use in support of the liver. By acting as an antioxidant, silymarin protects the liver and enhances the detoxification process. I highly recommend that any COPD patient with a history of smoking, who has been or is currently on prescription medication, and has had a less-than-optimal diet, be supplementing daily with milk thistle seed and lipotropic factors. This will provide your liver the support it needs to continue to efficiently act as your body's detoxifying organ. The efficacy of milk thistle seed is very well established in the scientific research literature.

Hydration and the critical role of water

One of the simplest and yet most effective ways to help with the mucus problem of COPD is to ensure that you drink enough water. By drinking water, I mean pure water, and not iced tea, lemonade, or whatever else you may be counting as water because it is made with water. I cannot tell you the number of people I know who believe that because they drink what they think are enough beverages that contain water, this counts as the water they are supposed to be drinking. Nothing could be further from the truth. In order for water to be effective, it has to be consumed in its pure form.

Most people are chronically dehydrated because of inadequate water intake. Digestive problems, compromised organ function, arthritis, bladder problems, obesity, diabetes, arteriosclerosis, kidney stones, and headaches are just a few of the health issues that are either related to or aggravated by inadequate water consumption. Your body is composed of approximately 70 percent water, which makes it one of the most important molecules in your body. If you do not consume enough pure water, many physiological functions will become compromised. Proper transport of nutrients throughout your body, blood circulation, efficient excretion of wastes and sweating, maintenance of blood pressure and body temperature, and a myriad of chemical reactions in your body are all dependent upon an adequate supply of water.

Specifically as it pertains to COPD, an adequate supply of water and proper hydration will help to reduce the viscosity of your mucus secretions. This will enable you to expectorate mucus with much greater ease and with less physical effort in coughing. This may sound too simple, but it is an absolutely proven fact that sufficient hydration will help in reducing the viscosity of mucus secretions from the respiratory tract. Despite its simplicity, however, this still remains an area where patient compliance leaves a lot to be desired.

You have probably learned that in order to maintain adequate hydration you should drink between eight and ten 8-ounce glasses of water a day. That would amount to a total of 64 to 80 ounces of pure water daily. This is a rather generic and arbitrary amount that takes no account of the specifics of your own body. A much more accurate and therapeutically beneficial way to calculate the amount of water you need to be drinking, especially to help in lessening the viscosity of mucus secretions, is a method based on your body weight. In order to maintain adequate hydration for essential bodily functioning, as well as helping to reduce mucus viscosity, you need to be drinking between ½ and ⅔ of your body weight in ounces of water per day. Let me show you how this is calculated. One half is 50 percent or .5. Two thirds is 66 per cent or .66. Just multiply your body weight by .5 and then multiply you body weight again by .66. Your answers will be a fraction (either .5 or .66) of your body weight in pounds, but what the numbers you derive are really telling you is the range of ounces of water you should be drinking daily. The following examples will demonstrate how these calculations are done so that you will always be able to determine the accurate amount of water you should be drinking on a daily basis as determined by your body weight.

Examples of calculating daily water intake:

100 pounds of body weight
100 x .5 = 50
100 x .66 = 66
Daily intake = 50–66 ounces

125 pounds of body weight
125 x .5 = 62.5
125 x .66 = 82.5
Daily intake = 63–83 ounces

150 pounds of body weight
150 x .5 = 75
150 x .66 = 99
Daily intake = 75–99 ounces

175 pounds of body weight
175 x .5 = 87.5
175 x .66 = 115.5
Daily intake = 88–116 ounces

200 pounds of body weight
200 x .5 = 100
200 x .66 = 132
Daily intake = 100–132 ounces

225 pounds of body weight
225 x .5 = 112.5
225 x .66 = 148.5
Daily intake = 113–149 ounces

16 ounces = 1 pint
64 ounces = 1 half-gallon

32 ounces = 1 quart
128 ounces = 1 gallon

You can see that the eight to ten 8-ounce glasses a day theory is only adequate for a 125-pound person. For persons lighter than 125 pounds, this amount would overhydrate them, which is not healthy either, and for persons over 125 pounds, this amount stills leaves them underhydrated. This is why you need to determine your daily water requirement based upon your body weight. The heavier you are, the more water you need. People who are dehydrated actually tend to retain water because their body is trying to compensate for the lack of water it receives. This contributes to obesity. If you are overweight, and you give your body the water it requires to carry out its metabolic business, you will find that you will not retain water, and you will actually begin to lose weight and start feeling much better.

As a final point, it is of the utmost importance to consider the quality of the water you are drinking. I highly recommend that under no circumstances should you ever drink tap water. Tap water is not safe and is deleterious to your health. Depending upon its source and method of treatment, municipal tap water may contain radon, fluoride, arsenic, iron, lead, copper, fertilizers, asbestos, cyanide, herbicides, pesticides, industrial chemicals, viruses, bacteria, parasites, chlorine, carbon, lime, phosphates, soda ash, or aluminum sulfate. It simply is not worth taking a chance by drinking tap water, especially when there are so many alternatives. I recommend drinking water that has been filtered by reverse osmosis. You can obtain bottled water that has been filtered in this manner, or you may purchase a unit that attaches to your sink. Commercially available filtering systems that use activated carbon are suitable as well. Bottled spring water can also be an acceptable choice as long as you are able to trust the source.

Final remarks

I encourage you to adopt the protocols outlined in this chapter as they will only bring benefit to your condition. You may be feeling some slight apprehension at present because of how drastic all these suggestions may appear to you. Unfortunately, your condition is rather serious, and despite the seemingly drastic nature of these dietary suggestions, they are necessary in order to get your condition under control and to get you headed in the right direction insofar as reestablishing your health is concerned. You have been given essentially every dietary and nutritional method that is currently known to help with COPD. Make use of the strategies given to the best of your ability and allow these nutritional methods to help you. No one expects you to adopt all of these protocols overnight. It may even take you several months until you have established yourself in your new dietary patterns, but the point is to work at it every day and see yourself making progress toward improving your condition. Once you begin to see the difference these dietary changes have made in your condition, you will be glad that you chose to make these changes.

Chapter 4

Nutritional Supplementation

Introduction

Nutritional supplements and herbs (herbs will be discussed in the next chapter on herbal medicine) will be two of the easiest protocols to assimilate because their manner of use is quite similar to the pharmaceutical medication you are already familiar with insofar as you are "taking pills or capsules" or "taking tinctures or liquid extracts." This similarity in the method of delivery, however, is where any similarity between supplements, or herbs, and pharmaceutical medications ends. To the extent that many of the supplements that will be recommended in this chapter are indicated for their ability to bring about specific symptomatic relief, they do not necessarily operate within the body in the same manner as pharmaceutical drugs. Supplements and herbs, although they may have a predominant action that enables them to be classified for a particular use, are usually multitasking in that while they do indeed perform their predominant function, they are often involved in many other biochemical reactions that are synergistically working together to improve the overall health of the individual. Pharmaceuticals have no such beneficial synergistic effect, and they are usually accompanied by the potential, if not definite consequence of undesired and adverse side effects, which is almost never the case with nutritional supplements when they are used properly. Nutritional supplements, when used as part of a complete and holistic program of care, are not only able to provide relief from the symptoms of COPD but they also participate in a myriad of other biochemical processes occurring within your body that are working toward reestablishment of your overall health.

Using nutritional supplements safely and effectively — nebulizer use

Nutritional supplements are just that — supplements. That is to say that they are to supplement, or complement, the primary therapeutic intervention of dietary and nutritional modification. Always continue to bear in mind that the cornerstone of health — and the key factor in addressing your COPD — is in implementing the protocols that were addressed in the last chapter on dietary and nutritional therapeutics. Let us recall that it is the underlying issue of chronic inflammation that gives rise to the constant production of mucus in the respiratory tract. Inflammation in the respiratory tract in and of itself is not experienced symptomatically, but what you do experience symptomatically on a regular basis are the consequences of inflammation: the constant accumulation of mucus that is always clogging up your respiratory tract and obstructing your airways, and the coughing that always accompanies the mucus. You can take medication or supplements to thin the secretions, thereby making them easier to expectorate, but if you don't concurrently address the issue of inflammation as well, you will always remain in an uphill battle insofar as this particular aspect of your problem is concerned. The point is this: Use the supplements recommended in this chapter, or the herbs that will be discussed in the next chapter, but only as an adjunct to an overall comprehensive program that is grounded in the dietary modifications discussed in chapter 3.

Although the natural and alternative methods presented in this book are designed to be used in concert with each other, it is always with the understanding that dietary and nutritional therapeutics are the foundation upon which all other therapeutic methods are built. I used the example of inflammation to illustrate the necessity for a holistic therapeutic approach that is grounded in dietary and nutritional modification, because in many ways, inflammation is central to many of the other problems associated with COPD. Within the context of a holistic therapeutic approach to addressing the issues of COPD, successfully addressing the underlying problem of chronic inflammation will make it much easier to lessen or eliminate the other problems that are associated with COPD.

Most of the supplements that will be introduced in this chapter will be taken orally, usually in pill or capsule form. Some of the supplements that will be introduced, however, are in liquid form, and these liquid supplements will either be taken orally or be inhaled via a nebulizer. Most of you are probably already familiar with a nebulizer unit as this is probably the way in which you take your albuterol or other bronchodilators. For those of you who are not familiar with a nebulizer setup, it consists of a small air compressor (usually smaller than a shoebox) that forces compressed air through a tube into a container (the nebulizer) that holds a small amount of liquid. The nebulizer is about the size of a shot glass, and it has a lid and two openings. The first opening is at the bottom of the nebulizer, and this is where the tube from the compressor attaches. The other opening is on the lid. When the compressed air from the machine passes through the nebulizer holding the liquid, it changes the liquid into a mist such that the mist passes through the opening on the lid of the nebulizer into another tube that goes to either a mouthpiece, a mask, or a tracheal mask in the event that the patient is a laryngectomee. The mist is then inhaled directly into the lungs over a period of five to twenty minutes, depending upon how much liquid was in the nebulizer, and this constitutes what is commonly known as a nebulizer treatment. This is a highly effective way to deliver appropriately indicated liquid supplements, herbal tinctures, and medications directly into the respiratory tract.

A quality home nebulizer unit can be bought on–line anywhere from $60.00 to $150.00. The nebulizer containers, masks or mouthpieces, and tubing will have to be replaced from time to time at nominal cost. From my own personal experience I recommend MisterNeb, Respironics, or Omron as quality affordable brands that you can trust. Allergy Be Gone is a reputable company in New York that carries all of these brands, and they are available to answer any questions you may have as well as providing information on the use, care, and cleaning of a nebulizer. Their contact information is listed in appendix 3. Figure 8 illustrates a complete nebulizer unit.

Figure 8 **Illustration of nebulizer compressor, tubing, nebulizer container, and mouthpiece.**

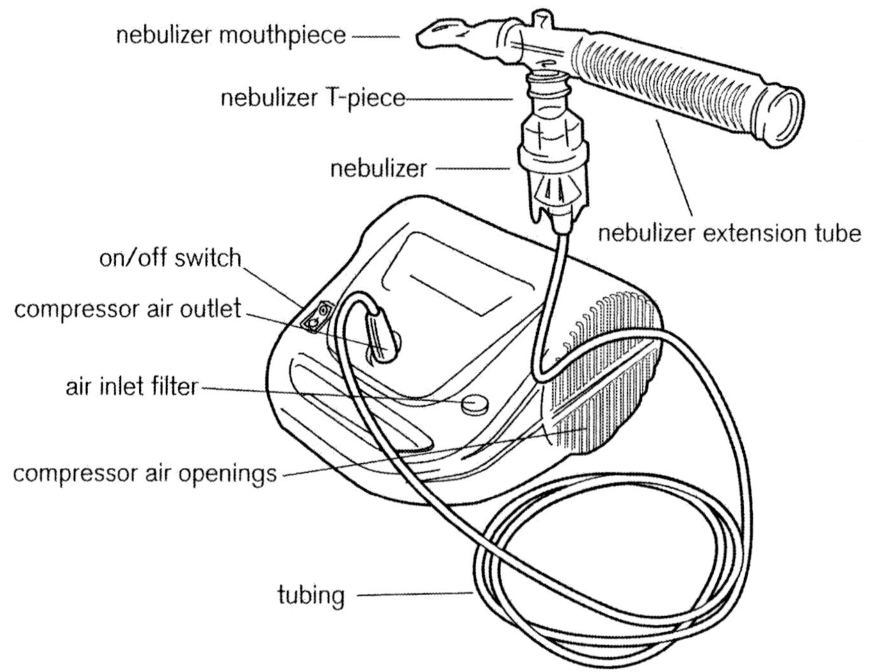

To ensure safety in using nutritional supplements, whether taken orally or via a nebulizer, always exercise responsibility and care in their administration. Never exceed dosage recommendations, and always give supplements their due respect. People often think that vitamins, supplements, or herbs are inherently safe because they are "natural." This is not always true. There are supplements and herbs that can be dangerous if they are mishandled or used inappropriately. As I have stated throughout this book, you should be working with a healthcare professional in the administration of the protocols from this book. This book is not a self-help guide in the sense that you are to be implementing these protocols entirely on your own without any guidance. COPD is serious and warrants professional care. This book is a guide to what can be done for your condition, and as such it is an educational tool for you and your physician, but the actual implementation of the protocols should always be under the guidance of your physician or healthcare provider.

Let us now begin our discussion of the supplements that are capable of addressing the issues of COPD. The supplements have been categorized according to the area where they demonstrate the greatest efficacy based upon research findings and/or clinical experience; however, some supplements with multiple actions will be listed in more than one category. Insofar as there are quite a few supplements that are going to be discussed, this does not imply that you should be using every supplement that is discussed in this chapter. The variety of choices that exists within some of the categories makes for the "gray area" that was discussed in the last chapter. As you may have several choices within any given category, it would be most prudent for you to be working with a healthcare professional who is not only familiar with the nuances of your case, but who is also sufficiently trained and possesses the necessary experience so as to be able to help you select the supplements that will benefit you most. The descriptions that follow will give you essential information about the supplement, any possible adverse reactions, if any, any contraindications or drug interactions with other substances you may be taking, and appropriate dosing amounts. The descriptions contain some scientific language that is necessary in order that healthcare professionals may better understand the scientific basis for why the particular supplement was recommended. By having a mechanistic understanding of the supplement's action, your healthcare provider can better assist you in the selection of supplements that are most appropriately suited for the particularities of your situation.

<u>Anti–Inflammatory Supplements</u>

1. Quercetin

Quercetin is a flavonoid. Food sources of quercetin are garlic, onions, green tea, grapefruit, and St. John's Wort. Research indicates that quercetin can function as an antioxidant, anti–inflammatory, antiviral, and an immunomodulator. In particular, as it pertains to its usefulness in COPD, quercetin exhibits anti–inflammatory properties through its ability to inhibit lipoxygenase, the enzyme necessary for the formation of pro–inflammatory leukotriene B_4 (LTB_4). (See figure 7 in chapter 3.) Research also indicates quercetin's ability to inhibit the formation of pro–inflammatory 2 series prostaglandins. Other studies have also shown that quercetin inhibits mast cells, basophils, and neutrophils, further substantiating quercetin's anti-inflammatory and immunomodulating activity. As quercetin's inhibition of lipoxygenase limits the formation of all 4 series leukotrienes, quercetin can also aid in lessening bronchoconstriction. The absorption of quercetin is believed to be enhanced by bromelain and papain.

<u>Adverse reactions</u>
Rare: Nausea, headache, and mild tingling in the extremities

<u>Contraindications and drug interactions</u>
Quercetin should not be taken by individuals who are currently taking quinolone antibiotics or cisplatin. Quercetin is capable of competitively inhibiting quinolone antibiotics and is also capable of causing toxicity in individuals using cisplatin. Quercetin should be avoided by pregnant women and nursing mothers.

<u>Dosage and administration</u>
Tablets or capsules: 500 milligrams, 3 times daily

2. Evening primrose oil

Evening primrose oil is obtained from the seeds of the evening primrose plant. As a rich source of omega–6 gamma–linolenic acid (GLA) and its precursor, linoleic acid (LA), evening primrose oil is able to reduce inflammation by significantly influencing the biochemistry of the eicosanoids. Through its conversion to dihomo–gamma–linolenic acid (DGLA), GLA reduces inflammation and lessens bronchoconstriction by competitively inhibiting the formation of 4 series leukotrienes and 2 series prostaglandins. When DGLA is metabolized to 15–hydroxyl DGLA, it blocks the conversion of arachidonic acid to 4 series leukotrienes, particularly LTB_4, thereby effectively reducing inflammation. Furthermore, DGLA is the precursor molecule to prostaglandin E_1 (PGE_1), which exerts an inhibitory effect on polymorphonuclear leukocytes. PGE_1 also increases intracellular levels of another cellular messenger molecule known as cyclic AMP (cAMP). An increased level of cAMP reduces the release of lysosomal enzymes, reduces leukocyte chemotaxis, and induces the relaxation of bronchial smooth muscle. As evening primrose oil is only a source of omega–6 GLA and LA, to get the full anti–inflammatory benefit available through essential fatty acid therapy, and to maintain a good balance between the omega–6 and omega–3 fatty acids, you should also supplement with flaxseed oil, which is an excellent source of omega–3 alpha–linolenic acid (ALA).

<u>Adverse reactions</u>
Possible: Nausea, vomiting, bloating, flatulence, and diarrhea

<u>Contraindications and drug interactions</u>
Pregnant women or nursing mothers should avoid evening primrose oil. Individuals with a history of seizure disorders or schizophrenia and individuals with hemophilia or who are taking warfarin (coumadin) should avoid evening primrose oil. If hempseed oil, supplemental garlic, ginkgo biloba, or fish oils are being used simultaneously with evening primrose oil, exercise care as these combinations may increase susceptibility to nosebleeds or bruising.

<u>Dosage and administration</u>
Capsules: 400–3,000 milligrams daily in divided doses

3. Flaxseed oil

Flaxseed oil is an excellent source of essential fatty acids as it is one of the few plants that contain both omega–3 and omega–6 fatty acids. Flaxseed oil consists mainly of omega–3 alpha–linolenic acid (ALA) and a moderate source of omega–6 linoleic acid (LA). As a rich source of alpha–linolenic acid (ALA), flaxseed oil exhibits its usefulness as an anti–inflammatory in COPD when ALA is metabolized to eicosapentaenoic acid (EPA), which is the precursor of the anti–inflammatory 3 series prostaglandins and 5 series leukotrienes. It is also believed that ALA may inhibit the formation of pro–inflammatory 2 series prostaglandins, leukotriene B_4, and pro–inflammatory cytokines. As a limited source of linoleic acid (LA), which can be converted into gamma–linolenic acid (GLA), flaxseed oil can also contribute to reducing inflammation through the anti–inflammatory actions of GLA as discussed in the previous section on evening primrose oil.

<u>Adverse reactions</u>
Possible: Diarrhea

<u>Contraindications and drug interactions</u>
Flaxseed oil should be avoided by pregnant women or nursing mothers. Individuals with hemophilia or who are taking warfarin (coumadin) should use flaxseed oil with caution. If hempseed oil, supplemental garlic, ginkgo biloba, or fish oils are being used simultaneously with flaxseed oil, exercise care as these combinations may increase susceptibility to nosebleeds or bruising.

<u>Dosage and administration</u>
Capsules: 1,000–6,000 milligrams daily in divided doses
Bottles of oil: Follow directions on label.

4. Hempseed oil

Hempseed oil is obtained from the seeds of the cannabis plant. Hempseed oil, however, contains essentially none of the psychoactive components of marijuana. Hempseed oil is sold as a nutritional supplement by several companies, and it is legal in all states. Hempseed oil is an excellent source of essential fatty acids as it is also one of the few plants that contain both omega–3 and omega–6 fatty acids. It has a natural nutty flavor that makes it very palatable. As a moderate source of omega–3 alpha–linolenic acid (ALA), hempseed oil's usefulness as an anti-inflammatory is partially due to the anti–inflammatory properties of ALA as discussed in the previous section on flaxseed oil. Hempseed oil is also a rich source of omega–6 linoleic acid (LA) as well as a moderate source of omega–6 gamma–linolenic acid (GLA). As a source of GLA, as well as LA, which is the precursor to GLA, hempseed oil exhibits the anti–inflammatory properties attributed to GLA as discussed in the section on evening primrose oil.

<u>Adverse reactions</u>
Rare: Nausea, diarrhea

<u>Contraindications and drug interactions</u>
Hempseed oil should be avoided by pregnant women and nursing mothers. Hempseed oil should be used with caution in persons with hemophilia or who are using the drug warfarin (coumadin). Hempseed oil should also be used cautiously in persons with diagnosed breast or prostate cancer. If flaxseed oil, evening primrose oil, supplemental garlic, ginkgo biloba, or fish oils are being used simultaneously with hempseed oil, exercise care as these combinations may increase susceptibility to nosebleeds or bruising.

<u>Dosage and administration</u>
Capsules or bottles of oil: Follow directions on label.

5. d – α – tocopherol (Vitamin E)

Vitamin E is well established as an antioxidant, which makes it quite useful in counteracting some of the effects of the oxidative damage that exists in the lungs. Vitamin E also has other clearly established health benefits that make it an appropriate supplement for general health maintenance. As it pertains to inflammation in COPD, there is scientific research to indicate that vitamin E and vitamin E analogs are inhibitors of phospholipase A_2. By inhibiting the release of arachidonic acid, vitamin E consequently lessens the formation of pro–inflammatory 4 series leukotrienes and 2 series prostaglandins. This implies that vitamin E can contribute to reducing the inflammation and bronchoconstriction associated with COPD.

<u>Adverse reactions</u>
None reported

<u>Contraindications and drug interactions</u>
Pregnant women, nursing mothers, or individuals taking warfarin (coumadin) or other anticoagulant drugs should use vitamin E with caution. Individuals with a history of hemorrhagic stroke, hemophilia, or vitamin K deficiency should use extreme caution with vitamin E. Vitamin E may enhance the antithrombotic activity of garlic and ginkgo biloba when used concurrently. Dietary fiber supplements and vitamin E supplements should be taken separately.

<u>Dosage and administration</u>
Tablets or capsules: 400 I.U., 3–4 times daily. Take with 50–100 milligrams of vitamin C. Higher doses of vitamin E may be needed for therapeutic benefit; however, do not exceed 1,600 I.U. daily without physician recommendation and supervision. Natural Vitamin E 400 I.U. by Solgar, in vegetarian softgels, is a good choice.

6. Inosine

Inosine is a purine ribonucleoside found in a variety of plant and animal sources. The popular use of inosine is as an endurance enhancer for athletes, a claim that may be due to the fact that inosine is a precursor molecule to ATP, which is the energy currency of the cell. There is no research evidence to support the use of inosine as an endurance enhancer; however, inosine does have significant research support as an anti–inflammatory and an immunomodulator. Inosine has been shown to inhibit pro–inflammatory cytokines to include tissue necrosis factor alpha (TNF–α), interleukin (IL)–1, interleukin (IL)–12, macrophage–inflammatory protein–1 alpha, and interferon (IFN)–gamma in cell culture studies of immunostimulated macrophages. On this basis, inosine clearly warrants consideration for use in addressing the inflammation associated with COPD.

<u>Adverse reactions</u>
Occasionally: Abdominal discomfort, nausea

<u>Contraindications and drug interactions</u>
Inosine should be avoided by pregnant women, nursing mothers, and individuals with a history of gouty arthritis. Individuals with a history of hyperuricemia should use extreme caution in using Inosine.

<u>Dosage and administration</u>
Tablets or capsules: 1,000–5,000 milligrams daily. Do not exceed 5,000 milligrams per day unless under the direction of a physician.

7. Zinc

As a divalent cation under physiological conditions, zinc is an essential element that is involved in a myriad of biochemical reactions. As it pertains to COPD, though, there is research to suggest that zinc ions (Zn^{2+}) can inhibit phospholipase A_2. Through inhibition of phospholipase A_2, zinc may contribute to lessening the release of arachidonic acid, which would then lessen the formation of pro–inflammatory 4 series leukotrienes and 2 series prostaglandins. This would result in reducing inflammation and bronchoconstriction. As an immune system enhancer, zinc is believed to stabilize cell membranes that are involved in signal transduction processes in cell–mediated immunity. By stabilizing immunological transcription factors, zinc may also influence gene expression.

<u>Adverse reactions</u>
Possible: Nausea, vomiting, metallic taste, headache, or drowsiness may occur at doses greater than 30 milligrams.

<u>Contraindications and drug interactions</u>
Quinolone antibiotics or tetracyclines taken concurrently with zinc may decrease the absorption of both the antibiotics and zinc. Pregnant or nursing mothers should not exceed 15 milligrams per day of zinc.

<u>Dosage and administration</u>
Tablets or capsules: 50 milligrams, 2–3 times daily. Zinc "50" by Solgar is a good choice.

8. Manganese

In similar fashion to zinc, manganese in its divalent form (Mn^{2+}) has research to suggest its use as an anti–inflammatory through its proposed ability to inhibit phospholipase A_2. The research to support both zinc and manganese as phospholipase A_2 inhibitors is limited; however, it is university-based basic science research that is conclusive in its findings. Based upon this research evidence, and the fact that zinc and manganese are not harmful supplements to use under normal conditions, there is no reason not to try and see if they will help in your particular case.

<u>Adverse reactions</u>
None reported

<u>Contraindications and drug interactions</u>
Individuals with hepatic disease, particularly liver failure, should not use manganese. Pregnant women or nursing mothers should not exceed 5 milligrams daily. The absorption of manganese may be decreased if manganese is taken concurrently with antacids, laxatives, tetracycline, calcium, iron, or magnesium.

<u>Dosage and administration</u>
Tablets or capsules: 2–10 milligrams daily

9. Bromelain

Bromelain is the name given to the group of proteolytic enzymes derived from the pineapple plant. Bromelain consists mainly of cysteine proteases along with lesser amounts of cellulase, peroxidase, amylase, and acid phosphatase. Bromelain's mechanism of action is not yet fully elucidated; however, research indicates bromelain's usefulness in COPD due to its anti–inflammatory and immunomodulatory properties. As a mucolyltic, bromelain has shown benefit in decreasing the viscosity of mucus secretions in chronic bronchitis. The activity of bromelain may be enhanced when combined with quercetin and vitamin C.

<u>Adverse reactions</u>
Occasionally: Vomiting, diarrhea, cramping, metrorrhagia, and menorrhagia

<u>Contraindications and drug interactions</u>
Bromelain should be avoided by pregnant women or nursing mothers. Bromelain should be used with caution in patients who are using anticoagulants or antithrombotic agents as bromelain may enhance the activity of these drugs. Bromelain has also been reported to increase the serum levels of amoxicillin and tetracycline when used concurrently. Bromelain should not be used by anyone with a known hypersensitivity to bromelain.

<u>Dosage and administration</u>
Tablets: 500–2,000 GDUs (gelatin digestion units), 1–3 times daily. Take bromelain on an empty stomach.

10.   Pycnogenol — See pycnogenol under *antioxidant supplements.*

11.   Grape seed extract — See grape seed extract under *antioxidant supplements.*

Mucolytic Supplements

1. N–Acetylcysteine (NAC)

The use of acetylcysteine in COPD is very well established in the scientific literature. Acetylcysteine acts as both an antioxidant and a mucolytic. L–cysteine, a major component of acetylcysteine, is one of the precursors of glutathione, a powerful antioxidant that will be discussed in the section on antioxidant supplements. As a mucolytic, acetylcysteine reduces disulfide linkages in the mucoproteins that comprise mucus, thereby effectively reducing the viscosity of mucus secretions. Acetylcysteine can be taken either orally in capsule or tablet form, or in liquid form via a nebulizer. NAC capsules or tablets are available as a nutritional supplement, whereas liquid acetylcysteine requires a prescription. There is variation in opinion as to which route of administration, oral or inhaled, is the most effective in exerting mucolytic effect in COPD. Both routes of administration may be used simultaneously with care. Follow the guidelines at the end of chapter 3 for the amount of water you need to be drinking as it is necessary to remain very well hydrated when taking acetylcysteine.

Adverse reactions
Possible: Nausea, vomiting, diarrhea, headache, and rashes

Contraindications and drug interactions
Pregnant women or nursing mothers should only use NAC under the supervision of a physician. Individuals with a history of peptic ulcer disease should use NAC cautiously. Individuals using nitrates may experience headaches if using NAC concurrently. NAC may reduce serum levels of carbamazepine in patients taking this drug.

Dosage and administration
Capsules or tablets: 600–1,200 milligrams, 1–3 times daily. Take on an empty stomach. Take with 50 milligrams of vitamin B_6 and 100 milligrams of vitamin C for better absorption.
10% or 20% solution: Follow orders from your physician

2. Bromelain — See bromelain under *anti–inflammatory supplements*.

Bronchodilator Supplements

1. Magnesium

Although the exact mechanism of action of magnesium as a bronchodilator is not fully understood, there is research and epidemiological data to support the use of magnesium in COPD. Magnesium has been demonstrated to relax smooth muscle, a finding that clearly indicates its potential usefulness as a bronchodilator. The relaxation of the smooth muscle surrounding the bronchi and bronchioles enables these airways to expand, which allows for greater airflow and ease in breathing.

Adverse reactions
Possible: Nausea, diarrhea. You can avoid these potential adverse reactions by taking magnesium with food.

Contraindications and drug interactions
Pregnant women and nursing mothers should not exceed 350 milligrams of supplemental magnesium daily unless directed by a physician. Magnesium should be avoided by individuals with renal failure or atrioventricular (AV) blocks. Individuals diagnosed with myasthenia gravis should also avoid supplemental magnesium.

Dosage and administration
Tablets or capsules: 350–500 milligrams daily. Use chelated form of magnesium. Take with 700–1,000 milligrams of calcium. Do not exceed 500 milligrams daily without consulting your physician.

<u>Antioxidant Supplements</u>

1. Vitamin C with bioflavonoids (to include rutin)

Vitamin C is clearly established as one of the most important antioxidants in existence. Vitamin C is capable of reducing reactive oxygen species (oxygen free radicals) as well as reactive nitrogen compounds. Vitamin C also helps to maintain cellular concentrations of reduced glutathione, another extremely important antioxidant. As an antioxidant, vitamin C protects the bronchial airways from oxidative stress that can lead to bronchoconstriction. Vitamin C is also helpful in protecting against the oxidative damage brought about through smoking. Vitamin C also enhances immune function, acts as an anti–inflammatory by reducing histamine levels, and aids in the healing of inflamed tissue. In helping to repair damaged lung tissue, vitamin C is involved in the biosynthesis of elastin, the principal protein molecule that comprises the elastic fibers within the interalveolar septum (alveolar wall).

<u>Adverse reactions</u>
Possible: Nausea, diarrhea, or flatulence. If any of these occurs simply cut back the amount of vitamin C and the problem should resolve.

<u>Contraindications and drug interactions</u>
Individuals on chemotherapy should consult their physician before taking supplemental vitamin C.

<u>Dosage and administration</u>
Capsules or tablets: 1,000 milligrams every 2–3 hours for a total of 6,000–10,000 milligrams daily. Use a buffered form of vitamin C that also contains calcium and magnesium for better absorption.

2. Glutathione

Glutathione is a tripeptide, synthesized mainly in the liver, which consists of the amino acids L–cysteine, glycine, and L–glutamate. Research to date has shown glutathione to be a powerful antioxidant that is well indicated for use in COPD. The majority of the body's glutathione supply is in the form of reduced glutathione, the feature that enables glutathione to function so effectively as a reducing agent. Through its ability to act as an intracellular redox buffer, glutathione is able to scavenge free radicals and keep other important antioxidant molecules such as vitamin C in their reduced state. Considering the significant amount of oxidative damage that exists within the respiratory tissue of smokers and COPD patients, glutathione is an important supplement whose therapeutic value cannot be emphasized enough. Research substantiates the ability of glutathione to be beneficial in reversing the oxidant–antioxidant imbalances that occur in lung tissue as a result of the oxidative stress and inflammation associated with COPD. Oral glutathione can be taken either as straight glutathione or as a combination of the three amino acids. Research findings are somewhat divided as to which method of taking oral glutathione is best absorbed. Insofar as there is enough evidence to suggest that oral intake of straight glutathione is poorly absorbed, it is sufficient to simply supplement with the individual amino acids L–cysteine, L–glutamate, and glycine. As long as you have a properly functioning liver, your body will make glutathione for you from these precursors. If you are taking oral acetylcysteine (NAC) to help with your mucus situation, you need not take any additional L–cysteine as this is already contained within NAC. Although oral supplementation of the glutathione precursors will be beneficial to you, the preferred manner of taking glutathione in the case of COPD is via a nebulizer. You will need to obtain I.V.-grade reduced glutathione, and this will require a prescription. Liquid glutathione is not readily available at just any pharmacy. It usually has to be made by a compounding pharmacist who understands how to properly prepare reduced glutathione for use in a nebulizer. If you have access to such a pharmacist and have a doctor who will write the prescription, then you are set. If, however, you lack these luxuries, I offer the following option as a convenience to you. Medaus Pharmacy, a compounding pharmacy in Birmingham,

Alabama, is well versed in making nebulizer-grade reduced glutathione. They have a referral network of physicians all over the United States that they work with regularly. If you call them and tell them the area where you live, they will refer you to the physician in their network that is closest to your area. Contact information for Medaus Pharmacy is contained in appendix 3. This way, you not only get your glutathione prescription but you meet a physician who is in all likelihood orientated toward natural and alternative medicine and may have the appropriate background to work with you. Upon receiving the prescription from the physician, Medaus will send you your supply of reduced glutathione for your nebulizer. In addition to just straight glutathione in the nebulizer, the following formula can also be used. This formula also requires a prescription because of the first three ingredients. If your physician orders this formula, Medaus will prepare the formula and then ship it to you. This outstanding comprehensive nebulizer formula has helped many COPD patients in ameliorating their symptoms and aiding in healing damaged lung tissue through its major actions as an antioxidant, anti–inflammatory, anti–bacterial/anti–viral, and an expectorant.

COPD NEBULIZER FORMULA

1.	I.V.-grade reduced glutathione	20 ml
2.	I.V.-grade vitamin C	8 ml
3.	I.V.-grade 0.9% normal saline	44 ml
4.	Glycyrrhizic acid (liquid extract)	20 ml
5.	Children's glycerite (liquid extract)	28 ml

Children's glycerite is a formula in and of itself that contains echinacea, wild black cherry bark, yerba santa, elecampane, goldenseal, osha, mullein, ginger, and bitter orange essential oil. In addition to being part of the COPD nebulizer formula, children's glycerite liquid extract can also be taken internally by itself as follows: mix 20–60 drops (1–2 ml) with a glass of water 1–4 times a day. Children's glycerite is safely tolerated when used in accordance with labeling instructions and is available through Wise Woman Herbals. Appendix 3 contains contact information for Wise Woman Herbals.

<u>Adverse reactions</u>
None reported

<u>Contraindications and drug interactions</u>
Pregnant women and nursing mothers should avoid supplemental glutathione unless under the direction of a physician. Ensure adequate water consumption when taking either glutathione or the amino acid precursors.

<u>Dosage and administration</u>

<u>Straight glutathione</u>
Capsules or tablets: 600 milligrams daily

<u>Amino acid combination</u>
Capsules or tablets:
L–cysteine: 500–1500 milligrams daily (only if not using NAC)
L–glutamate (glutamic acid): 100–500 milligrams daily
Glycine: 500–1000 milligrams daily in divided doses

<u>Nebulizer glutathione</u>
Follow prescribing instructions from physician.

<u>COPD NEBULIZER FORMULA</u>
1–2 ml every 3–4 hours as needed (physician dosing guidelines)

3. Selenium

Selenium's main function as an antioxidant is through the role it plays, along with vitamin E, in the formation of glutathione peroxidases. The selenium-dependent glutathione peroxidases play significant roles in preventing oxidative damage to cell membranes and eliminating peroxides in the extracellular fluid. Insofar as COPD patients have much more oxidative damage to their lungs than nonsmokers, and are at higher risk for lung cancer, by reducing the concentrations of reactive oxygen in cells, particularly those of the respiratory epithelium, the glutathione peroxidases play a key role in regulating signal transduction pathways and protecting DNA from oxidative damage.

<u>Adverse reactions</u>
None within the dosing range indicated

<u>Contraindications and drug interactions</u>
Pregnant women and nursing mothers should not exceed 400 micrograms daily.

<u>Dosage and administration</u>
Capsules or tablets: 50–400 micrograms daily. Up to 900 micrograms daily may be taken under the guidance of a physician.

4. Pycnogenol

Pycnogenol is the name given to the class of antioxidant compounds known as procyanidins that are derived from the French maritime pine. Research suggests pycnogenol's ability to act as an anti–inflammatory is due to its antioxidant capacity to scavenge reactive oxygen and nitrogen species, as well as superoxide radicals, hydroxyl radicals, lipid peroxyl radicals, and peroxynitrite radicals. Research also seems to indicate that pycnogenol inhibits the activation of several transcription factors that upregulate some of the cytokine inflammatory mediators. Pycnogenol has also been shown to specifically inhibit smoking-induced platelet aggregation as well demonstrating protection against the tobacco-specific nitrosamine, NKK.

<u>Adverse reactions</u>
None reported

<u>Contraindications and drug interactions</u>
Pregnant women and nursing mothers should avoid supplemental pycnogenol.

<u>Dosage and administration</u>
Capsules or tablets: 200 milligrams daily

5. Grape seed extract (proanthocyanidins)

In similar fashion to the pycnogenol just discussed, grape seed extract proanthocyanidins, otherwise known as OPCs, are also of the class of procyanidins that have strong antioxidant and anti–inflammatory properties. Additionally, grape seed extract may also have anticarcinogenic activity as there is research that has demonstrated grape seed extract's ability to significantly inhibit lung cancer in the laboratory.

<u>Adverse reactions</u>
None reported

<u>Contraindications and drug interactions</u>
Pregnant women and nursing mothers should avoid grape seed extract.

<u>Dosage and administration</u>
Capsules or tablets: 50–200 milligrams daily

6. d – α – tocopherol (vitamin E) — See vitamin E under *anti–inflammatory supplements.*

Other Useful Nutrients/Supplements for COPD

1. Lactoferrin (antibacterial)

Lactoferrin is a 703 amino acid containing glycoprotein that is part of the iron transporter family. Through its ability to strongly bind iron, which is essential for the growth of pathogenic bacteria, lactoferrin inhibits pathogenic bacterial growth. Lactoferricin, a bioactive metabolite of the breakdown of lactoferrin, in addition to exhibiting antibacterial action, exhibits antiviral action as well due to its ability to inhibit viral cell fusion and the entry of viruses into normal cells.

Adverse reactions
None reported

Contraindications and drug interactions
Pregnant women and nursing mothers should avoid lactoferrin.

Dosage and administration
Capsules: 250 milligrams daily

2. Chlorophyll/chlorophyllin, green food (detoxification)

Consumption of green drinks should be part of the daily regimen of every COPD patient. Research clearly indicates chlorophyll's usefulness as a detoxifying agent, antimutagenic, and anticarcinogenic. Chlorophyllin has demonstrated the ability to inhibit several mutagens, including those found in cigarette smoke and coal dust. *Greens for Life* by Formulations for Life is an excellent green food supplement in powder form that is mixed with water or juice. In addition to its content of many green vegetables, *Greens for Life* also contains milk thistle, bromelain, grape seed extract, quercetin, and probiotics, all of which are very important for an individual with COPD. Supplemental chlorophyllin is available in capsule or liquid form.

Adverse reactions
Possible: Discoloration of urine or feces may occur, although this is nothing to worry about.

Contraindications and drug interactions
Pregnant women and nursing mothers should consult with a physician before using chlorophyll/chlorophyllin supplements.

Dosage and administration

Chlorophyll (*Greens for Life*)
Powder: Follow instructions on label.

<u>Chlorophyllin</u>
Capsules or liquid: Follow instructions on label.

3. **Multivitamin/multi–mineral complex** (overall health)

Daily consumption of a multivitamin/multi–mineral complex is an essential for every COPD patient. The main issue at hand with a multivitamin is which one to take, as there are so many to choose from. Quality and formulation are the key things to look for, and I urge you not to compromise on either of these two factors. Pure Encapsulations Nutrient 950 is one of the best multivitamin/multi–mineral complexes available. The only problem is that Pure Encapsulation products are not available for sale to the general public. You can only obtain Pure Encapsulation products from a healthcare professional who has an established relationship with the company. Among companies that manufacture multivitamin/multi–mineral complexes that are available for sale to the general public, Solgar, Twinlab, Solaray, or Natrol are good choices.

<u>Adverse reactions</u>
See label for any adverse reactions.

<u>Contraindications and drug interactions</u>
See label for any contraindications or drug interactions.

<u>Dosage and administration</u>
Capsules or tablets: Follow instructions on label.

4. **B-complex vitamins** (tissue repair and healing)

The B vitamins serve as cofactors for over 100 enzymes. In order that these enzymes may perform their functions, many of which involve healing and tissue repair, an adequate amount of B vitamins is necessary. B–complex "100" by Solgar is an excellent choice.

<u>Adverse reactions</u>
See label for any adverse reactions.

<u>Contraindications and drug interactions</u>
See label for any contraindications or drug interactions.

<u>Dosage and administration</u>
Capsules: Follow instructions on label.

5. Superoxide dimutase (antioxidant)

Superoxide dimutase (SOD) is the name given to a class of enzymes that are involved protecting cells from oxidative damage. SOD neutralizes free radicals, particularly the superoxide radicals, by converting them into hydrogen peroxide and molecular oxygen. The ability of SOD to neutralize superoxide radicals, which are the most common free radicals in the body, is beneficial in addressing the oxidative damage in lung tissue. SOD is measured in terms of McCord–Fridovich (MF) units.

<u>Adverse reactions</u>
See label for any adverse reactions.

<u>Contraindications and drug interactions</u>
See label for any contraindications or drug interactions.

<u>Dosage and administration</u>
Tablets: 2000 MF units, 1–3 times daily in between meals

6. Colloidal silver (anti–infective)

Silver is well established as an antimicrobial agent. Colloidal silver has been subjected to conventional university-based research as well as substantial testing in independent laboratories, and is considered to be one of the most universal antimicrobial substances known. Its use was part of mainstream medicine until the advent of patented antibiotics in the 1940s. Silver has the capability of killing hundreds of microorganisms, including MRSA, a capability that no modern antibiotic can match. The exact mechanism of action of colloidal silver is still to be fully elucidated; however, it is believed that colloidal silver acts by disabling the enzymes that pathogenic microorganisms are dependent upon. Bacterial microorganisms, in particular, do not develop a resistance to silver as they do to antibiotics. There are many brands of colloidal silver on the market, and they are not all equal. Most brands are mainly composed of silver ions, and silver ions are not true colloidal silver. Brands made of a high silver ion content may contribute to the development of argyria (a condition where the skin turns blue/gray due to exposure to certain forms of silver). True silver colloids (true colloidal silver) will not cause argyria, and they have the highest ratio of pure silver colloids to effectively destroy pathogenic microorganisms. Mesosilver, made by Purest Colloids in New Jersey, is widely regarded as one of the best colloidal silver products available on the market today, and the only form of colloidal silver that I use personally. Mesosilver can be taken internally or via a nebulizer.

<u>Adverse reactions</u>
None. Argyria only occurs with ionic silver or silver protein products. True colloidal silver should not cause argyria.

<u>Contraindications and drug interactions</u>
Pregnant women or nursing mothers should check with their physician before using colloidal silver. Individuals who are allergic to silver should avoid using colloidal silver.

<u>Dosage and administration</u>
Liquid colloidal Mesosilver: For infection prevention, the dosage for Mesosilver is typically one teaspoon (5 ml) daily as follows: 3 ml to be taken internally and the other 2 ml to be taken via nebulizer. For use during an acute stage of infection, take 5 ml internally and 5 ml via nebulizer every 3–4 hours until the infection abates.

Table 7 on the next page is a generalized summary of the nutritional supplements for COPD that have been discussed in this chapter.

Table 7

Nutritional Supplements Summary

Anti–Inflammatory

1.   Quercetin
2.   Evening primrose oil
3.   Flaxseed oil
4.   Hempseed oil
5.   d–α–tocopherol
     (vitamin E)
6.   Inosine
7.   Zinc
8.   Manganese
9.   Bromelain
10. Pycnogenol
11. Grape seed extract

Mucolytic

1.   N–Acetylcysteine
2.   Bromelain

Bronchodilator

1. Magnesium

Antioxidant

1. Vitamin C
2. Glutathione
3. Selenium
4. Pycnogenol
5. Grape seed extract
6. d–α–tocopherol
   (vitamin E)

Other Supplements

1. Lactoferrin
2. Chlorophyll/
   chlorophyllin
3. Multivitamin/
   multi–mineral
4. B complex vitamins
5. Superoxide dimutase
6. Colloidal silver

Chapter 5

Herbal Medicine

Introduction

Herbs have been an integral part of the healing arts since the dawn of civilization. For thousands of years now, essentially every known culture that has ever inhabited the planet Earth has used herbs medicinally. Although herbs have an extensive history of medicinal use, there are still a few individuals within the mainstream medical establishment that either frown upon their use or just outright dismisses their medicinal worth. These individuals will usually defend their position toward herbs by asserting that herbs are not "scientifically proven" to be effective. Nothing could be further from the truth, and, once again, perspective is everything.

The truth of the matter is that the medicinal properties of herbs have been "proven" when you broaden the criteria of what is accepted as the standard of proof. In today's scientific and technologically driven world of medicine, the standard of proof for medicinal efficacy has been narrowed to the point where only the information that is derived through conventional scientific research and controlled double–blind studies is considered acceptable. Conventional scientific research is usually aimed at attempting to explain the mechanism of how a substance works fundamentally, while double–blind studies attempt to determine whether or not the substance under investigation is clinically effective and safe for use in human beings. Although current research methods are absolutely necessary in order to advance our understanding of science and medicine, and double–blind studies certainly yield much-needed data concerning a substance's clinical efficacy and safety, I would contend that it would be very remiss of us to disregard the wisdom and knowledge of medicinal herbs that has been formulated by various cultures throughout history if it is only for the reason that many of these herbs have not been subjected to current research protocols or double–blind studies.

There are many drugs that are routinely used in medicine today that may have "passed" the criteria of double–blind studies, yet the mechanism of how they work fundamentally is still not known. Not fully understanding how a drug works, however, does not necessarily stop modern medicine from using the drug. But what is to be said of the "proof" that is derived through the history of a substance being used safely and effectively for hundreds or thousands of years? I would submit that if an herb has been consistently and reliably used over the centuries because of its recognized and effective medicinal properties, then this in and of itself establishes the basis of historical "proof." I would further submit that using the historical record of an herb to substantiate its medicinal value is every bit as legitimate as a modern double–blind study. Passing the test of history, rather than a clinical trial, is what has enabled us to know how to use any particular herb safely, effectively, and appropriately.

It is encouraging to know that over the last two decades since the American public began to undergo a paradigm shift in their perceptions towards healthcare and began to embrace natural approaches to maintaining their health, the medicinal use of herbs has experienced a tremendous renaissance that is still flourishing to this day. The paradigm shift that has been occurring across America has been not only driven by a culminating dissatisfaction with the conventional healthcare system's limitations to effectively address the myriad of health issues that confront a significant portion of the American population, but also because America has slowly and steadily become aware that the true key to addressing chronic disease lies in embracing and applying the principles and methods of natural medicine and the natural approaches to health and living. The vast majority of the American public has now come to realize that natural medicine is a very viable means by which to improve their health, and the number of skeptics within the conventional healthcare system toward the use of medicinal herbs is rapidly diminishing.

In most cases the medicinal use of herbs today is still based upon their historical use, however, the herbal medicine renaissance that has been growing in America over the last couple of decades has provided the impetus for the scientific research of herbs that is now occurring in many of our university research laboratories. Much of what is being discovered through the scientific analysis and research of herbs is confirming what has been known empirically throughout history. Research is also resulting in the discovery of new applications and roles that herbs play in human health. The significant benefit of this research though, is that it has begun to present scientific explanations for the actions of herbs, which provides the credibility and justification required by the conventional medical community to substantiate their use.

Unlike pharmaceutical medications, which are single isolated compounds, herbs contain many compounds. Although only some of the compounds within an herb may be responsible for giving the herb the medicinal attributes for which it is classified, you must understand that these "active ingredients" of the herb are working synergistically within the context of the larger molecular population of the whole herb that was assembled by nature. Many of the conventional drugs that are used in mainstream medical practice today are isolated derivatives of herbs. When you isolate a compound from an herb and manufacture it as a single drug, you take that compound out of its natural context, and not only do you then lose synergy but you invite all the side effects and complications that result from using an isolated compound that is not in its natural form. Aspirin is an easy example to make this point. As far back as the fifth century B.C., willow bark was known for its ability to reduce fever and relieve pain. It wasn't until the 1800s, some 2,200 years later, that salicin, the active extract of the willow bark, was isolated and crystallized. The salicin that is contained within willow bark is what you have come to know as aspirin. It is not that aspirin is inherently bad in and of itself; it's the notion that nature intended for salicin to exert its action within the context of the whole herb. Willow bark, when used to relieve pain or reduce fever, has no side effects. Willow bark may take a little longer to begin acting, but its effect may actually last longer, and unlike aspirin, it doesn't cause bleeding in the stomach or have an association with a more serious health concern such as Reye's Syndrome. Herbs, in general, are obviously not without their potential side effects, but when properly administered, the potential side effects of herbs are usually rare and significantly less serious than the common, and very often deleterious, side effects of pharmaceutical medications.

It is interesting to note that the vast majority of serious illness in this country is all lifestyle related. Heart disease, cancer, stroke, and COPD (the top four leading causes of death in the United States) are all for the most part diseases of lifestyle. There is the occasional unfortunate case where one of these illnesses has struck an individual who otherwise lived a healthy life, but by and large these are diseases that are intrinsically rooted in our dietary habits and our lifestyle choices. We are as critically ill as we are because of the bad choices we have made, and if we weren't so sick as a result of our bad choices, we wouldn't need such aggressive medication to help us stay alive. Fortunately, though, Americans have begun to realize these things, and along with beginning to embrace natural alternatives to their healthcare, they have more importantly begun to really understand diet and nutrition as the cornerstone of health and are making the necessary changes in their eating habits so as to avert serious disease and live healthier, happier, and longer lives.

Herbs can't cure everything. The fact is that herbs don't cure anything — your body is the only thing that can cure itself. Herbs, however, like supplements and other natural health methods, when given an optimal environment in which to work that is predicated upon proper dietary and nutritional modifications, are remarkably effective at helping the body along in its quest to heal itself. On the pages that follow, you will become acquainted with the specifics of how herbs can be used to help with COPD. The herbs that are useful for addressing the issues of COPD and building up your health are abundant. I encourage you to take full advantage of the rich herbal tradition that has served humanity throughout the centuries.

The use of herbs in COPD

The value of herbs as part of a complete holistic approach to address the issues of COPD is incalculable. Within the context of an approach that is always grounded in the dietary and nutritional approaches that were covered in chapter 3, not only can herbs be used to address the main symptomatic issues of COPD, but they also work synergistically to help bring about overall healing and restoration of health to the extent that is possible. I continue to repeat the underlying theme of dietary and nutritional modification because this is the single most important aspect of your entire healing process. I always want you to remember that everything you do (supplements, herbs, exercise, etc.) to help with your health is secondary to changes you need to make in your diet.

The realm of herbal medicine is vast, and the choices you have amongst the variety of herbs to use for COPD are numerous. The forty-five different herbs that have been chosen for inclusion in this chapter all have a well–established historical basis for their use in COPD. In the next section of this chapter titled "single herbs for COPD," you will find a collection of monographs, each of which gives a detailed description of the twenty-four herbs that I consider to be the most important for addressing the various issues related to COPD. Although these herbs usually have multiple actions that synergistically work together, I have only indicated those actions that are immediately relevant to COPD. Within these monographs you will be introduced to herbs that have demonstrated efficacy as immune system enhancers; anti–infectives, to include antivirals, antibacterials, and antimicrobials; expectorants to help with clearing the respiratory passages of mucus; antioxidants to address the oxidative damage to the lungs and to assist with healing; and anti–inflammatories that work to reduce inflammation, bronchoconstriction, and mucus formation. In every monograph, the historical use of the herb is always given, and in most cases, the findings of current scientific research are also discussed to further substantiate the action and uses of the herb.

All of the herbs that are discussed in the monographs, with the exception of olive leaf, are indicated to be used orally as a liquid extract. Olive leaf is indicated to be used orally as a capsule only because the capsule form is the most readily available form of olive leaf. The liquid extract form is indicated for every other herb because liquid extracts are easier to assimilate than capsules. By using liquid tinctures, you minimize any issues that you may have in assimilating the herb in the event that you have less than optimal absorption as a consequence of intestinal problems. Oregano oil liquid extract, in addition to being used orally, can also be used via a steam inhalation device or a nebulizer.

Working with herbs can take some getting used to at the beginning, but eventually it can become an enjoyable process, especially when it comes to using bulk herbs to prepare the formulas for the herbal tea combinations. Using herbs, whether as liquid extracts or teas, is an area where you are going to have a fair degree of choice in your selections. In similar fashion to finding which of the available dietary and juicing choices works best for your situation, you may find that you and your healthcare practitioner also have to experiment for a while before you find which herbs or combinations of herbs work best for the unique circumstances of your situation. This is one of the reasons why I have indicated forty-five different herbs overall and given ten different herbal tea combinations. Echinacea, ginger, licorice, and marshmallow all have anti–inflammatory properties, but in your case you may find that it is marshmallow in particular that provides you with the best results in helping with your inflammation. All of the herbs discussed in this chapter exert action according to their described properties; however, you may have to try several before finding which one exerts that action most effectively in you. This phenomenon is not unlike conventional drugs. There are many instances where several prescriptions have to be tried before finding one that "works." With herbs, though, when you find the ones that work, you not only get symptomatic relief, but you also gain the overall health benefits that result from the restorative energy and synergistic qualities of the herb.

Learn as much as you can about herbs. They are going to be an important factor in your healing process. In some respects herbs could have also been discussed under the heading of diet and nutrition because they are, after all, "food." When we think of herbs we often forget that as "plant foods" they also provide a whole spectrum of nutritional value that is also complementary to the healing process. Mark Pedersen's *Nutritional Herbology* is one of the few books that I have seen where a complete nutritional profile (vitamins, minerals, carbohydrates, proteins, fat, etc.) is given for many of the commonly used herbs. *The Herb Book*, by the renowned American naturopath John B. Lust, is a classic paperback compendium of essentially every

American herb known. Although many advancements have been made in our knowledge of herbs in the last thirty-one years since its publication in 1974, it is still one of the greatest herbals ever written and it is a great way to introduce yourself to the world of herbs. A great source for information on herbs and botanical medicine is the American Botanical Council (ABC). The American Botanical Council is a nonprofit, member–supported organization whose mission is to provide education using science–based and traditional information to promote responsible use of herbal medicine — serving the public, researchers, educators, healthcare professionals, industry, and the media. Contact information for the American Botanical Council can be found in appendix 3.

As you now begin to examine the specifics of the herbs that are useful in COPD, keep the following in mind. As I have mentioned over and over again in this book, you need to be working with a healthcare professional that is experienced in the methods of natural health. This will ensure not only that you have the appropriate oversight needed for your care, but that you also have the proper guidance in working with herbs. Working with a skilled practitioner who not only knows the nuances of your condition but who is also well versed in the use of herbs will in all likelihood enable you to determine the herbs that will benefit your condition in much less time. Also note the following conversion factor when determining dosages: 1 ml is approximately 28 drops.

<u>Single Herbs for COPD</u>

1. Astragalus

Properties: Immune system enhancer, antiviral, antioxidant
Part used: Dried root
Description: Astragalus is useful in COPD as it is effective in fighting infections of the mucous membranes, especially the mucous membranes of the respiratory tract. Astragalus is also an excellent tonic for strengthening the lungs and for the debility and wasting that often

accompany COPD. Astragalus has also been shown to inhibit lipid peroxidation, making it useful as an antioxidant.

Cautions: Do not use astragalus if you have a fever.

Method of use: Liquid extract taken internally by mouth

Dosage: 1–2 ml mixed with 4 ounces of water, 3–4 times daily

2. Cayenne

Properties: Expectorant, stimulant, antibacterial

Part used: Ripe fruit

Description: Cayenne pepper is useful as an expectorant in helping to expel the thick mucous secretions that are characteristic of COPD. Cayenne decongests the lungs and acts as a stimulant to enhance blood circulation. Because of its ability to enhance circulation, cayenne is often added to other herbs to enhance their absorption and effectiveness. Cayenne also contains compounds called capsaicinoids, and research has found that capsaicinoids have antimicrobial effects against streptococcus pyogenes. This enables cayenne to be very useful in addressing some of the respiratory tract infections, mainly pharyngitis and pneumonia, which often confront individuals with COPD.

Cautions: None when used as indicated

Method of use: Liquid extract taken internally by mouth

Dosage: 1 ml mixed with 4 ounces of water or juice, 3–5 times daily

3. Echinacea (purpurea and angustifolia)

Properties: Anti–inflammatory, immune system enhancer, collagen protection

Part used: Fresh root, leaves, and flowers

Description: The use of echinacea is very well warranted for COPD. Research substantiates echinacea as an anti–inflammatory through its ability to inhibit both cyclooxygenase and 5–lipoxygenase (see figure 7, chapter 3). By inhibiting cyclooxygenase and 5–lipoxygenase, echinacea effectively reduces the formation of pro–inflammatory 4 series leukotrienes and 2 series prostaglandins. This will contribute to lessening the inflammation in the bronchial walls, help open the airway, and reduce mucus production. Research has also shown that echinacea enhances the ability of polymorphonuclear leukocytes to kill staphylococci. This is an important capability of echinacea insofar as many COPD patients have tested positive for MRSA (methicillin–resistant staphylococcus aureus), an antibiotic-resistant strain of staphylococci. Staphylococcus aureus is oftentimes the pathogenic culprit involved in the recurrent episodes of pneumonia that are experienced by individuals with COPD. Because of staphylococcus aureus' resistance to antibiotics, an episode of pneumonia due to staphylococcus aureus can be particularly serious for a COPD patient. Echinacea should therefore always be considered in the treatment strategy for a staphylococcus aureus–related infection. Echinacea also contains caffeic acid derivatives known as echinacosides. These compounds have been shown to protect type III collagen from the damage caused by oxygen free radicals. This makes echinacea important in helping to maintain the structural integrity of the acinus and promoting the healing of damaged tissue, as type III collagen is a constituent of the interalveolar septum.

Cautions: None when used as indicated

Method of use: Liquid extract taken internally by mouth

Dosage: 2 ml mixed with 4 ounces of water, 3–6 times daily. In cases of severe infection, up to 4 ml every 1–2 hours may be used until the infection abates.

4. Elecampane

Properties: Expectorant, respiratory tonic, antibacterial

Part used: Dried root and flowers

Description: Elecampane is useful for the excessive mucous secretions that constitute the wet, productive coughs that are often characteristic of chronic bronchitis. Elecampane is cleansing and tonifying to the mucous membranes of the respiratory tract. The sesquiterpene lactones contained in elecampane have demonstrated antimicrobial and antifungal activity.

Cautions: Pregnant women should avoid elecampane.

Method of use: Liquid extract taken internally by mouth

Dosage: 1–2 ml mixed with 4 ounces of water, 3–5 times daily

5. Garlic

Properties: Antimicrobial, antiviral, antioxidant, lipid–lowering
Part used: Fresh whole bulb
Description: The usefulness of garlic as a natural antibiotic against staphylococcus and streptococcus is well established in the scientific literature. There is also research to indicate garlic's ability as an antiviral. Garlic has antioxidant properties insofar as it has been shown to increase intracellular levels of reduced glutathione. Amongst its many medicinal uses, garlic has been used historically for infections, inflammation, and clearing mucus in the respiratory tract. Although not directly related to COPD, garlic's well–established ability to lower total serum cholesterol, and LDL–C (low–density lipoprotein cholesterol) in particular, is a positive health benefit not to be ignored.
Cautions: Pregnant women or nursing mothers should consult with their physician before using garlic. Use cautiously if taken concurrently with evening primrose oil, flaxseed oil, hempseed oil, vitamin E, ginkgo biloba, or anticoagulant drugs such as coumadin. Garlic may also cause abdominal upset in some individuals.
Method of use: Liquid extract taken internally by mouth
Dosage: 2 ml mixed with 4 ounces of water or juice, 2–3 times daily

6. Ginger

Properties: Anti–inflammatory, carminative, diaphoretic, expectorant
Part used: Dried root
Description: Ginger is traditionally used for its well–established ability to aid digestion and to relieve nausea, vomiting, indigestion, and gas. Research has shown that ginger also acts as an anti–inflammatory, and it is thought that ginger's action as an anti–inflammatory is through the inhibition of 5–lipoxygenase and cyclooxygenase. Through the inhibition of these enzymes, ginger acts to reduce the formation of 4 series leukotrienes and the pro–inflammatory 2 series prostaglandins. With a reduction in leukotrienes and pro–inflammatory prostaglandins, there will be a consequent reduction of inflammation and bronchoconstriction.

Ginger has also been used as an expectorant, and to relieve shortness of breath.

Cautions: None when used as indicated

Method of use: Liquid extract taken internally by mouth

Dosage: 1–2 ml mixed with 4 ounces of water or juice, 3–4 times daily

7. Ginkgo biloba

Properties: Anti–inflammatory, antioxidant

Part used: Fresh leaves

Description: Although Ginkgo biloba is best known for its ability to enhance peripheral blood circulation, its primary usefulness in COPD stems from its ginkgolide B content. As a strong inhibitor of platelet–activating factor (PAF), ginkgolide B blocks PAF from binding its receptor. By blocking the binding of PAF, the ginkgolide B in ginkgo inhibits the bronchoconstriction and airway hyperactivity that is induced when PAF is allowed to bind its receptor. The flavonoid compounds in ginkgo also contribute to ginkgo's anti–inflammatory properties by reducing neutrophil infiltration. As an antioxidant, ginkgo acts as a free radical scavenger and also inhibits lipid peroxidation.

Cautions: Use ginkgo cautiously when taken concurrently with evening primrose oil, flaxseed oil, hempseed oil, vitamin E, garlic, or anticoagulant drugs such as coumadin.

Method of use: Liquid extract taken internally by mouth

Dosage: 1–2 ml mixed with 4 ounces of water, 3–4 times daily

8. Ginseng (Siberian and American)

Properties: Rejuvenating tonic, antioxidant, antiviral

Part used: Dried root

Description: As COPD is most often an affliction of the middle–aged to the elderly, ginseng is quite useful in addressing the debility that is associated with COPD and aging. Ginseng strengthens the lungs and enhances both physical energy and mental acuity. Ginseng exhibits antioxidant properties through its ability to increase hepatic glutathione peroxidase activity. There is also research to suggest that ginseng can stimulate cell-mediated immunity.

Cautions: Do not use ginseng if you have a fever, or during an acute infection. Individuals with heart disease or diabetes should consult with their physician before using ginseng.

Method of use: Liquid extract taken internally by mouth

Dosage: 1–2 ml mixed with 4 ounces of water, 2–3 times daily

9. Goldenseal

Properties: Anti–inflammatory, antibacterial

Part used: Dried root

Description: The drying and cleansing effect that goldenseal has on mucous membranes makes it useful in addressing the chronic inflammation and bronchial phlegm that is characteristic of COPD. Goldenseal has also been shown to be effective against streptococcus pyogenes and staphylococcus aureus. This ability makes goldenseal, like echinacea, particularly useful in addressing the staphylococcus aureus–related infections such as pneumonia that often beset COPD patients who are positive for MRSA (methicillin–resistant staphylococcus aureus). A combination of the extracts of echinacea and goldenseal, when used prophylactically, can be an effective preventative measure against the myriad of pathogens that are involved in the recurrent respiratory infections seen in COPD.

Cautions: Goldenseal should be avoided by pregnant women and individuals with glucose–6–phosphate dehydrogenase deficiency. Goldenseal should only be used for a week or two at a time as it can weaken the intestinal flora.

Method of use: Liquid extract taken internally by mouth

Dosage: 1–2 ml mixed with 4 ounces of water, 3–4 times daily

10. Grindelia (gumweed)

Properties: Expectorant, antibacterial, anti–inflammatory

Part used: Dried leaves and flowers

Description: Grindelia can be useful in COPD for bronchial irritation, and with unproductive coughs that are associated with wheezing and constricted airways. Grindelia is also useful for upper respiratory tract

infections, as it has been shown that grindelia has both antibacterial and antimicrobial activity. Grindelia also has demonstrated anti–inflammatory action.
Cautions: None when used as indicated
Method of use: Liquid extract taken internally by mouth
Dosage: 1–2 ml taken with 4 ounces of water, 2–4 times daily

11. Horehound

Properties: Expectorant, anti–infective
Part used: Dried leaves and flowers
Description: Horehound is traditionally used for respiratory catarrh, which is inflammation of the respiratory mucous membranes that is accompanied by an increase in mucus flow. Because of its chlorogenic acid content, horehound is also capable of exhibiting broad-acting antiviral and antibacterial activity.
Cautions: Horehound is not to be used during pregnancy
Method of use: Liquid extract taken internally by mouth
Dosage: 1–2 ml mixed with 4 ounces of water or juice, 3–4 times daily

12. Hyssop

Properties: Expectorant, anti–infective
Part used: Fresh or dried leaves and flowers
Description: Hyssop has been historically used for mucous congestion in the lungs. Hyssop also contains compounds that are antimicrobial and antiviral.
Cautions: Pregnant women should avoid hyssop.
Method of use: Liquid extract taken internally by mouth
Dosage: 1–2 ml mixed with 4 ounces of water, 2–3 times daily

13. Licorice

Properties: Anti–inflammatory, antiviral, expectorant
Part used: Dried root
Description: The anti–inflammatory and antiviral properties of licorice are well researched and established. Licorice exhibits anti– inflammatory

action through several different mechanisms to include inhibition of cyclooxygenase and lipoxygenase. Inhibition of these enzymes will result in reducing the formation of 4 series leukotrienes and 2 series prostaglandins, which will lead to a reduction of the inflammation and bronchoconstriction in the bronchial wall. As an antiviral, licorice is effective against influenza infection, a feature that is clearly beneficial for COPD patients. Licorice is soothing to the mucous membranes of the respiratory tract and is useful in clearing the phlegm associated with chronic bronchitis.

Cautions: Pregnant women should avoid licorice. Individuals with liver disease, diabetes, high blood pressure, and heart disease should consult with their physician before using licorice. Excessive, long–term use of licorice can result in high blood pressure; however, any elevation in blood pressure due to use of the herb will return to normal when use of the herb is stopped.

Method of use: Liquid extract taken internally by mouth

Dosage: 1–2 ml mixed with 4 ounces of water, 3–4 times daily

14. Marshmallow

Properties: Anti–inflammatory, expectorant, antioxidant

Part used: Fresh root

Description: Marshmallow is very soothing to the mucous membranes of the respiratory tract. It is particularly indicated when bronchial irritation and inflammation is associated with a dry, less productive cough. Marshmallow also exhibits strong antioxidant activity through its ability to scavenge superoxide anion radicals.

Cautions: None when used as indicated

Method of use: Liquid extract taken internally by mouth

Dosage: 2–3 ml mixed with 4 ounces of water, 3–4 times daily

15. Milk thistle

Actions: Antioxidant, protects liver

Part used: Dried seed

Description: Milk thistle is necessary for individuals with COPD due to the increased demands placed on the liver as a result of the oxidative stress that is a consequence of COPD. This means that extra care should be taken to protect the liver of an individual with COPD because of all the extra work the liver has been subjected to by having to detoxify all the toxins found in cigarette smoke, a poor diet, and prescription medications to name a few. Silymarin, one of the main compounds in milk thistle, exerts a wide variety of liver-protecting properties through its actions upon both hepatocytes (liver cells), and Kupffer cells, which are specialized macrophages within the liver. Silymarin protects liver cells from toxins and decreases the production of nitric oxide and superoxide anion radicals by Kupffer cells. Although nitric oxide and superoxide anion radicals serve a limited purpose as part of the macrophage's process of killing pathogens, and are otherwise relatively harmless in and of themselves, these free radicals can lead to undesired oxidative damage because they can readily react to form other free radicals, such as hydroxyl radicals, which are very dangerous to cells. Silymarin also inhibits the formation of leukotrienes by Kupffer cells, which helps to reduce inflammation in the liver. Silymarin increases the liver's production of the all-important antioxidant glutathione, and silymarin also enhances the regenerative ability of the liver. Considering the central role the liver plays as the body's major detoxifying organ, milk thistle is an important herb for COPD.

Cautions: None when used as indicated

Method of use: Liquid extract taken internally by mouth

Dosage: 1–2 ml mixed with 4 ounces of water or juice, 2–3 times daily

16. Mullein

Actions: Anti–inflammatory, expectorant

Part used: Fresh leaves, flowers, and root

Description: Mullein, in similar fashion to marshmallow, is very soothing to the mucous membranes of the respiratory tract. Mullein eases inflammation and has an expectorant effect on the phlegm associated with chronic bronchitis.

Cautions: None when used as indicated.

Method of use: Liquid extract taken internally by mouth

Dosage: 2–3 ml mixed with 4 ounces of water, 3–4 times daily

17. Myrrh

Actions: Anti–inflammatory, expectorant
Part used: Resin from the bark
Description: Although myrrh is best known as an ingredient used in making incense, its medicinal use for COPD is well substantiated. Myrrh is particularly useful in cases of chronic bronchitis where the mucous membranes have become sluggish and there is excessive and persistent mucus, or in cases of bronchiectasis where oftentimes you have green sputum that is indicative of stagnant pus. Whether it is from chronic inflammation or infection, whenever there is excessive and tenacious mucus in the respiratory tract, myrrh should always be considered as part of the therapeutic protocol.
Cautions: Pregnant women should avoid myrrh.
Method of use: Liquid extract taken internally by mouth
Dosage: 1–2 ml mixed with 4 ounces of water, 2–4 times daily

18. Olive leaf

Actions: Antiviral, anti–inflammatory
Part used: Dried leaves
Description: Herbalists know olive leaf for its effectiveness as a broad-spectrum antiviral and antibacterial. Olive leaf extract, which contains the compound oleuropein, possesses the natural ability to inhibit the growth of numerous viruses, bacteria, and other pathogens. Olive leaf extract has been shown to be effective against flu and colds, bacterial infections, allergies, hepatitis B, and hepatitis C, to name a few. Olive leaf also contains several flavonoids, most of which have demonstrated anti–inflammatory activity. As COPD patients are often prone to respiratory infections and/or pneumonia, olive leaf should always be one of the first herbs of choice in the therapeutic intervention against infections.
Cautions: None when used as indicated
Method of use: Capsules (standardized extract) taken internally by mouth
Dosage: 1–2 capsules with water, 2–3 times daily. Dosage may be increased in cases of severe infection under the guidance of a healthcare professional.

19. Oregano

Actions: Anti–infective, anti–inflammatory, expectorant
Part used: Essential oil (Nature's Answer alcohol–free extract)
Description: The essential oil of oregano contains the compound carvacrol, which has demonstrated antimicrobial properties. This enables oregano to be helpful with some of the respiratory infections that are often troublesome for people with COPD. Oregano is useful for helping with the inflammation in the mucous membranes of the bronchial passages, and, as an expectorant, oregano is also useful in helping to clear the bronchial passages of mucus.
Cautions: None when used as indicated
Method of use: Liquid extract taken internally by mouth, steam inhalation, or inhalation via a nebulizer
Dosage: By mouth: ½ ml (14 drops) mixed with 2 ounces of water, 1–2 times daily. **Steam inhalation**: 1 ml (28 drops) mixed with 2–3 ounces of very hot (but not boiling) water in a steam inhaler, 1–2 times daily. The Vicks® Vaposteam® Inhaler is a good choice for a compact yet effective and inexpensive steam inhalation device. **Nebulizer:** ¾ ml (21 drops) mixed with 2 ml of warm distilled water, 1–2 times daily. Do not exceed a total of 2½ ml (70 drops) daily without consulting your healthcare professional.

20. Osha

Actions: Anti–infective, anti–inflammatory, expectorant
Part used: Root
Description: Osha is a traditional remedy with a long history of use in Native American medicine for respiratory conditions and inflammation. Osha root has expectorant, anti–infective, and anti–inflammatory properties that make it particularly useful for COPD. It is well suited for most infections of the respiratory tract, especially those that are viral in origin. It is effective for bronchial inflammation and helps bring up respiratory mucous secretions. By also acting to relax bronchial smooth muscle, osha helps to ease breathing by lessening bronchoconstriction. Osha also induces sweating and helps eliminate toxins through the pores of the skin.

Cautions: Pregnant women should avoid osha.
Method of use: Liquid extract taken internally by mouth
Dosage: 1–2 ml mixed with 4 ounces of water, 3–4 times daily

21. Thyme

Actions: Expectorant, antibacterial, bronchial antispasmodic
Part used: Leaves and flowers
Description: Thyme is useful in alleviating the bronchial spasms that are often associated with the coughing that is characteristic of COPD. Thyme is also quite useful for the catarrh of the upper respiratory tract that is commonly associated with COPD. Thyme exerts an expectorant effect on the cilia of the respiratory tract and can also be used as an antibacterial agent.
Cautions: None when used as indicated
Method of use: Liquid extract taken internally by mouth
Dosage: 1–2 ml mixed with 4 ounces of water, 3–4 times daily

22. Valerian

Actions: Sedative
Part used: Dried root
Description: The difficulties with breathing and the shortness of breath that a COPD patient experiences are often accompanied by anxiety, nervousness, and excitability. It is important, especially during an episode of acute dyspnea, to relax and remain calm while efforts are taken to ease your breathing. Valerian is a well–known sedative herb that can help with the anxiety you may have. Valerian can also be used to help with any restlessness that may be interfering with you getting a good night's sleep. Valerian contains valerenic acid, a compound that slows the degradation of the neurotransmitter GABA. By inhibiting the breakdown of GABA, valerian acts to help maintain appreciable levels of GABA in the synapse. It is believed that through increasing the availability of GABA, valerian has its sedative properties.
Cautions: Pregnant women should avoid valerian.
Method of use: Liquid extract taken internally by mouth
Dosage: 1–2 ml mixed with 2 ounces of water as needed

23. Wild cherry

Actions: Antitussive, sedative
Part used: Bark
Description: Wild cherry can help to calm the nerves that innervate the bronchial passageways. This can help to alleviate episodes of excessive and spasmodic coughing that often occur with COPD. Do not use wild cherry when the cough is productive, though, as this type of cough is helping to clear the bronchial passageways of mucus.
Cautions: None when used as directed
Method of use: Liquid extract taken internally by mouth
Dosage: ½ –1 ml mixed with 4 ounces of water, 2–3 times daily

24. Yerba santa

Actions: Expectorant
Part used: Dried leaves
Description: Yerba santa is used mainly for chronic bronchitis as an expectorant to help clear the bronchial passages of phlegm. It can be particularly useful in this manner when combined with grindelia.
Cautions: Pregnant women should avoid yerba santa.
Method of use: Liquid extract taken internally by mouth
Dosage: 1 ml mixed with 4 ounces of water, 2–3 times daily

Herbal Tea Combination Formulas for COPD

Herbal teas have a long history of use in medicine. Herbal teas not only provide you with a direct medicinal benefit, but they are also quite enjoyable, and they will serve as an excellent substitute for coffee or black tea. The formulas that follow are combinations of herbs to be prepared as an infusion and then drunk as a tea. I would suggest obtaining the herbs in bulk, prepare the formulas according to the ratios given, and then store each formula in a labeled mason jar such that they are readily available for your use. These bulk herbs can be obtained through Mountain Rose Herbs (see appendix 3). The following list is inclusive of all the herbs needed to make all of the tea formulas.

1. Anise seed
2. Chamomile
3. Elder flowers
4. Elecampane
5. Fennel seed
6. Flaxseed
7. Horsetail
8. Lavender
9. Licorice root
10. Lungwort
11. Marshmallow leaf
12. Marshmallow root
13. Mullein
14. Nettle leaves
15. Peppermint
16. Plantain
17. Sage
18. Thyme
19. Valerian
20. Wild cherry
21. Yarrow

Elecampane, flaxseed, fennel, licorice root, sage, valerian, and yarrow are not to be used during pregnancy.

Formulations that are soothing to the bronchial passageways and contribute to healing lung tissue

Formula 1

Marshmallow root	1 part
Licorice root	1 part
Flaxseed	2 parts

Infuse 1 teaspoon of formula 1 in a cup of boiling water. Sweeten with honey if necessary. Use up to 3 times daily.

Formula 2

Anise seed	1 part
Licorice root	1 part
Plantain leaves	1 part
Fennel seed	1 part

Infuse 1 teaspoon of formula 2 in a cup of boiling water. Sweeten with honey if necessary. Use up to 3 times daily.

Formula 3

Licorice root	1 part
Marshmallow root	1 part
Marshmallow leaf	1 part
Mullein	1 part

Infuse 1 teaspoon of formula 3 in a cup of boiling water. Sweeten with honey if necessary. Use up to 4 times daily.

Formula 4

Thyme	1 part
Elecampane root	1 part
Nettle leaves	1 part
Lungwort	1 part

Infuse 1 teaspoon of formula 4 in a cup of boiling water. Sweeten with honey if necessary. Use up to 4 times daily.

Formulations that are helpful for congestion, inflammation, and cough

Formula 5

Mullein	1 part
Lungwort	1 part
Plantain leaves	1 part

Infuse 1 teaspoon of formula 5 in a cup of boiling water. Sweeten with honey if necessary. Use once daily.

Formula 6

Lungwort	2 parts
Yarrow flowers	1 part
Plantain leaves	4 parts
Nettle leaves	2 parts

Infuse 2 teaspoons of formula 6 in a cup of boiling water. Sweeten with honey if necessary. Use once daily.

Formula 7

Nettle leaves	1 part
Horsetail	1 part
Lungwort	2 parts
Plantain leaves	2 parts

Infuse 3 teaspoons of formula 7 in a cup of boiling water. Sweeten with honey if necessary. Use once daily.

Formula 8

Yarrow flowers	4 parts
Lungwort	2 parts
Marshmallow root	1 part
Sage	1 part
Plantain leaves	2 parts

Infuse 1 teaspoon of formula 8 in a cup of boiling water. Sweeten with honey if necessary. Use up to twice daily.

Formula 9

Mullein	4 parts
Elecampane root	4 parts
Sage	1 part
Elder flowers	4 parts
Peppermint leaves	1 part
Wild cherry bark	4 parts
Thyme	4 parts

Infuse 3 teaspoons of formula 9 in a cup of boiling water. Sweeten with honey if necessary. Use up to 3 times daily.

Formulation that is calming and a sedative

Formula 10

Valerian root	2 parts
Chamomile flowers	1 part
Peppermint leaves	1 part
Lavender flowers	1 part
Yarrow flowers	3 parts
Fennel seed	3 parts

Infuse 1 teaspoon of formula 10 in a cup of boiling water. Use once daily.

Other Herbs to Consider

These herbs, to varying degrees, may also prove to be useful in addressing the issues related to your COPD.

Aloe vera	Antibacterial, antiviral, anti–inflammatory Taken as a juice
Bilberry	Anti–inflammatory, antimicrobial Taken as a tea
Cat's claw	Anti–inflammatory, antiviral Taken as a liquid extract
Eucalyptus	Expectorant, anti–inflammatory, antibacterial Taken as a tea by using the leaves Taken by steam inhalation when using the oil
Fenugreek	Expectorant Taken as a tea
Lobelia	Expectorant, bronchial spasms Taken as a liquid extract
Red clover	Expectorant, antispasmodic Taken as a liquid extract
Slippery elm	Expectorant, protects mucous membranes Taken as a tea

Aloe vera, cat's claw, fenugreek, and lobelia are not to be used during pregnancy.

Chapter 6

Exercise and Physical Therapeutics

Introduction

Physical activity is an essential part of maintaining health in general, and when it comes to building up the health of an individual with COPD, exercise and physical therapeutics should always be performed to the extent that an individual can tolerate. The sedentary lifestyle that often accompanies COPD will ultimately contribute to a deterioration in functional capacity, cardiovascular function, and skeletal muscle mass. In order to avoid further health complications that can result from a sedentary lifestyle, it is essential for you to maintain aerobic fitness and strength to the extent that you are able. Unlike therapeutic protocols such as diet and nutrition, nutritional supplements, and herbs, the degree to which a COPD patient can become involved with exercise or physical therapeutics will always depend upon the status of their condition. Many COPD patients are elderly, and perhaps fragile or debilitated, and these are factors that will limit the extent to which they can be involved with exercise or physical therapeutics.

The primary aim of exercise and physical therapeutics as it directly relates to COPD is to help you improve your breathing, help restore functionality, increase your vitality, and improve your quality of life. Exercise or physical therapeutics will not reverse any of the damage of COPD, but exercise will enable your muscles to adapt so as to be able to extract oxygen from the blood more efficiently. Once that adaptation has occurred, you will experience less shortness of breath upon exerting yourself. Exercise and physical therapeutics consist of activities such as walking and other aerobic exercise, pursed-lip breathing, diaphragmatic breathing, yoga, qigong, tai chi, and massage therapy. Although yoga, qigong, and tai chi are commonly performed in a group setting under the guidance of an experienced instructor, once you learn the techniques you can perform these activities alone at home. Massage therapy always needs to be done with a practitioner. Remember to consult with your physician before you commence any exercise program or utilize any of the modalities of physical therapeutics.

Walking and other aerobic exercise

Daily walking is one of the best exercise activities for a COPD patient. Walking will help your circulation and increase your stamina, and it will help build activity tolerance. Start out by walking half a block or less. Every other day, you should increase your walking distance a little bit. After a few months, you could be walking up to a mile without gasping for air. While you are walking, you should inhale through your nose and exhale through your mouth using the pursed-lip breathing technique. Pursed-lip breathing is discussed in the next section. Other aerobic forms of exercise that have a positive effect on COPD are treadmill walking, bicycling or stationary cycling, and swimming. As many daily activities also require the use of the arms and the upper body, it is advisable to include endurance and strength training for your upper body in your exercise program. Consult with your physician or physical therapist to find out what types of endurance or strength training are most appropriate for your situation.

Pursed-lip breathing

Pursed-lip breathing is one of the easiest ways to control episodes of breathlessness. This technique is a quick and easy way to slow down your pace of breathing so as to make each breath more effective. Pursed-lip breathing helps to prolong exhalation, which then helps to slow down your breathing rate. Pursed-lip breathing also helps to improve the ventilation of the lungs, keeps the airways open longer, and decreases the work of breathing. All of these factors contribute to easing your shortness of breath and helping you to relax. You can perform pursed-lip breathing as follows: While relaxing your shoulders and your neck, inhale (take a normal breath) slowly through your nose while keeping your mouth closed. Then purse your lips (position your lips) as you would if you were going to whistle. Slowly and gently exhale through your pursed lips. After you learn this technique with a little practice, you may utilize this technique whenever you find yourself having shortness of breath. Always make sure that your exhalation phase (breathing out) is longer than your inhalation phase (breathing in), and if you are using pursed-lip breathing while engaged in an activity, always make sure you are exhaling during the strenuous part of the activity.

Diaphragmatic breathing

Diaphragmatic breathing helps your lungs expand so that they take in more air. This breathing technique will help to strengthen your diaphragm as well as help to decrease the work of breathing by slowing down your breathing rate. When you practice this breathing technique, keep your chest, shoulders, and neck as relaxed as possible. The aim is to keep your upper body still and rely solely on your diaphragm. Diaphragmatic breathing is performed as follows: Lie on your back on a flat surface, such as the floor or your bed, with a pillow under your knees and your head. Your knees should be slightly bent. Place your left hand on your upper chest and your right hand on your abdomen. This will enable you to feel your diaphragm move as you breathe. With your hands in place as just described, inhale slowly through your nose so that your stomach moves out against your right hand. You should be able to feel your right hand on your abdomen moving out. Your left hand on your chest should not move at all. Then tighten your stomach muscles and let them move back in as you exhale with the pursed-lip technique. As you are exhaling, you should be able to feel your right hand on your abdomen moving in, and your left hand on your chest should still not be moving at all. After you have perfected diaphragmatic breathing while lying down, you can then do it while relaxing in a chair, or even standing. Diaphragmatic breathing should be practiced for 5–10 minutes, 3 to 4 times a day. Bending forward at the waist while breathing may also make it easier for you to breathe. As bending allows the diaphragm to move more easily, bending forward while breathing may help decrease shortness of breath, even with individuals who have severe COPD. You may bend forward while doing pursed-lip breathing or diaphragmatic breathing if you are sitting or standing.

Yoga

As far as the physical therapeutic techniques that have direct value for COPD, yoga, one of the oldest health practices in the world, gets my highest endorsement. Do not be dissuaded by any association that yoga may have with "new age." There are aspects of yoga that could be said to cross over into the spiritual arena, but as long as you remind yourself that you are utilizing yoga for its exercise benefit, and not for spiritual reasons, you can avoid any potential conflicts with any present spiritual or religious position that you hold. Your primary reason for doing yoga as a COPD patient is because yoga offers some of the best postural and breathing exercises in existence. The postures, or asanas, of hatha-yoga are excellent ways to develop strength and flexibility, which are very beneficial to an individual with COPD. Secondly, and perhaps a bit more importantly, though, are the breath-control techniques (pranayama) that can make a significant difference in enabling a COPD patient to breathe easier and develop exercise tolerance. Yoga is a completely holistic system of health practice that not only benefits both general and respiratory health but also reduces COPD-related stress and emotional duress through the promotion of relaxation and psychological stability. Individuals with COPD may find it helpful to begin yoga with breath-control (pranayama) exercises that can help strengthen the respiratory muscles, which will result in more control over breathlessness. This will increase your readiness for asana practice as well as other forms of exercise. Some of the simple yoga techniques can even aid individuals with advanced COPD. More information on yoga, as well as information on finding a yoga practitioner or instructor, can be obtained through the International Association of Yoga Therapists. Contact information for IAYT can be found in appendix 3.

Qigong and tai chi

The discussion of qigong and tai chi could have appeared in the next chapter under acupuncture and oriental medicine as both of these practices involve activating the energy that flows along the meridian pathways of the body. They are being discussed here, however, because they are modalities that are centered in physical exercise and the coordination of breathing. Tai chi is a form of qigong, and both of these modalities have their origin in the ancient healing systems of China. Both qigong and tai chi combine physical movement (exercise) and breath control so as to promote strength, increased flexibility, relaxation, and overall healing. Specifically as it pertains to COPD, the effects of practicing qigong or tai chi are similar to that of yoga. The physical exercises and breath control techniques will aid in reducing breathlessness and will lead to an overall increase in exercise tolerance. Qigong and tai chi will also stimulate immune function and improve circulation. Like yoga, qigong and tai chi are holistic systems of promoting health that, in addition to being able to address some of the symptomatic issues of COPD, will also help you greatly improve your overall health and wellness.

Massage therapy

Massage therapy is well indicated for use in respiratory disease. Massage therapy techniques used for COPD include postural drainage, manipulation of respiratory muscles combined with chest percussion, soft-tissue manipulation and joint mobilizations, and breathing exercises. When used as an adjunct therapy for COPD, massage therapy can help decrease shortness of breath, strengthen the muscles of respiration, improve forced vital capacity, reduce heart rate, increase oxygen saturation in the blood, and improve overall pulmonary functioning. Massage therapy can also help with other problems caused by COPD such as decreased rib cage mobility and neck problems. Because COPD patients often utilize the accessory muscles of respiration in their neck in order to get oxygen to the lungs, these muscles in the neck become overtaxed as they work to compensate for the lack of normal movement in the rib cage. Although massage therapy has its specific therapeutic benefits for

COPD, because it is also applied for the purpose of positively affecting your overall health and well being, it can be regarded as a welcome natural holistic complement for both your general health as well as addressing the issues of your COPD. For more information on massage therapy as well as finding a practitioner, contact the American Massage Therapy Association. Their contact information is in appendix 3.

Chapter 7

Other Alternatives and Considerations

Homeopathy

Homeopathy is probably one of the most misunderstood yet most potentially valuable therapeutic tools in the natural health arsenal. As always, though, this premise hinges upon the foundation of proper dietary and nutritional habits. Successful use of homeopathy involves not only the appropriate selection of a remedy, but also removing what are known as "obstacles to cure." The use of the word "cure" is not meant to infer that emphysema or COPD are curable, but rather that in order for homeopathy, or any other natural health protocol for that matter, to have maximum potential for effectiveness, obstacles such as a poor diet, smoking, or any other health-jeopardizing habits that would impede the process of healing must be eliminated.

There are many natural health books on the market today that will categorically list various homeopathic remedies to be used for the many different symptoms that are associated with emphysema or chronic bronchitis. There are books that will tell you to take belladonna when you have a dry cough that is accompanied by a fever and headache, hepar sulphuris when you have excessive mucus and coughing, or byronia when you have wheezing along with a fear of suffocation. Some books also suggest that natrum sulphuricum, aconite, phosphorus, aspidosperma, and carbo vegetabilis can be useful for one reason or another in addressing the problems with emphysema or chronic bronchitis. Depending upon how many books you look through, you could end up finding a litany of remedies being recommended to address the symptoms of COPD.

I personally feel it is irresponsible to recommend a homeopathic remedy based on only a couple of symptoms, especially when dealing with a chronic illness. People have somehow been inadvertently misled about how homeopathy works, and as a result they often do not have positive results with the remedies that they try, especially when they are trying to address issues involved with chronic disease. People may read something where it says to try this remedy for this or that symptom, or maybe they try a remedy based on the two or three symptoms indicated on the label of the remedy itself, but this is not how to do homeopathy. You don't select a remedy on just a couple of symptoms. You may have some success occasionally with selecting a proper remedy in this manner when dealing with an acute illness, but when it comes to chronic disease, you cannot just pick a remedy based upon a couple of symptoms. In fact, for the most part, a true constitutional homeopath wouldn't even prescribe for an acute illness just based on only two or three symptoms. Let me end this paragraph by making it absolutely clear that there are no homeopathic remedies for emphysema or COPD. There are remedies for you, an individual who happens to manifest the symptom picture of COPD, but there are no remedies for emphysema or COPD. Allow me to explain this.

If you want to be able to use homeopathy successfully in your attempts to rebuild your health, and to minimize or alleviate your COPD-related symptoms to the extent that it is possible, then you absolutely must work with a well-trained and skilled homeopathic practitioner. You cannot under any circumstances expect to have any real success if you attempt to do homeopathy alone. There are many reasons for this. It's not so much that homeopathy isn't safe to do alone, it's the fact that it takes a skilled practitioner to be able to find the right remedy that is appropriate for you.

Homeopathy is energetic medicine. That is to say that it does not act upon your body in the same mechanistic way as do drugs, or supplements, or herbs. One way in which this could be explained is to say that supplements, herbs, or drugs work within your body according to the laws of chemistry. They work in ways that involve physical interactions between molecules and cells. Homeopathic remedies, however, work on a whole different plane. You could think of homeopathy as being more in the realm of physics rather than chemistry. Although the mechanism of how homeopathy works is still not understood completely, homeopathy has nonetheless enjoyed great clinical success for over 200 years.

Homeopathy was developed by the German physician Samuel Hahnemann in the early nineteenth century. Due to his disgust with many of the toxic and deleterious medical practices of his day, Hahnemann sought to discover a means of healing that was more in accordance with natural laws. Hahnemann set about to find a way to firmly establish in clinical practice what had been known since 400 B.C. as the *law of similars*. Simply stated, the *law of similars* says that a remedy can cure a disease if it produces in a healthy person symptoms similar to those of the disease. Hahnemann conducted what are known as "provings," whereby he and other healthy willing subjects would ingest a substance in order that all the symptoms produced by ingesting that substance could be recorded. This was done for dozens and dozens of substances, and it ultimately resulted in what is known as the *Materia Medica*, which is a book that contains all the information about the symptoms that were elicited by all these different substances. In order to then "prove" the remedy, a minute dose of the remedy was given to a sick individual according to the *law of similars*, and in most cases the patient got well.

This is why it is so important for you to only do homeopathy with a skilled practitioner. In a typical initial appointment with a homeopathic practitioner, you are going to spend about an hour and a half just answering questions about all manner of things. This is because your immediate COPD symptoms are only part of a larger picture of you. Symptomatically speaking, there is a lot more going on underneath the surface than you would imagine. It is important to have a very comprehensive picture of the entirety of all the nuances that are related to you and your condition because all these nuances play a role in enabling the practitioner to select the appropriate remedy. Your main complaint may be excessive mucus and shortness of breath, but to the homeopathic practitioner, it is also important to know about your sleep habits, whether or not you prefer hot or cold beverages, whether or not your congestion is worse at night or in the morning, or whether or not you feel better outside in the fresh air or indoors. These are but a few of the many questions that are necessary in order to establish a complete picture of what remedy you are, but they are worth taking the time to answer because it enables the practitioner to best match the remedy according to the *law of similars*. The more information the practitioner has, the more accurately he or she can match your "profile" with the appropriate remedy. The appropriate remedy is going to be the substance that produced the same symptom picture in a healthy person that you are experiencing as a sick person.

To attempt to try to explain how it is that homeopathic remedies actually work would go beyond the scope of this book. As I previously mentioned, homeopathic remedies can be thought of more as a phenomenon of physics rather than chemistry. The answer clearly lies in the realm of physics and energy because there is no known pharmacological mechanism that can account for homeopathy's action. Because the remedies clearly exert action of clinical significance, the elucidation of the mechanism of how homeopathic remedies work is an active area of research amongst many physicists today. The remedies themselves are extremely dilute versions of the original substance that was tested in the original proving. So dilute are some of the remedies that there are no molecules of the original substance left in the solution. How can something have a medicinal effect if there are no molecules of it in the solution? The answer lies in the water and the potentization process. Potentization is part of the process of preparing a remedy whereby the substance undergoes a series of dilutions and succussions (vigorous shaking). We know that this process changes the energetic character of the water because we have nuclear magnetic resonance (NMR) studies that have conclusively shown that water that has undergone the homeopathic potentization process is clearly different from control water. How it all works and how it exerts its action on a biological system, though, is still an active area of investigation.

The main precept of this section has been to let you know that homeopathy can be very useful in helping you with your COPD, but that it is ill advised for you to attempt to treat yourself with homeopathic remedies. Homeopathic remedies are completely safe, but in the absence of a complete and thorough constitutional intake done by a professional practitioner, you will in all likelihood not select the right remedy that can help you. Homeopathy cannot cure emphysema or COPD, but when the appropriate remedy is selected, homeopathy can play a significant role in helping with reducing inflammation and shortness of breath, strengthening immunity, increasing your vitality, and improving your overall health. Appendix 3 contains information on how to find a skilled homeopathic practitioner.

Acupuncture and Oriental medicine

Acupuncture has been an integral component of traditional Chinese medicine for over 5,000 years. In addition to acupuncture, traditional Chinese medicine also has its own complete system of herbal medicine. Although Chinese immigrants brought acupuncture to the United States in the mid-nineteenth century, it did not establish itself as a distinct form of healthcare in this country until about thirty years ago, and it has only been in the last seven or eight years that acupuncture finally gained recognition from the mainstream medical community as a viable means of treatment for a variety of health conditions. Acupuncture's reputation, though, amongst the American public has been somewhat limited in that it is mainly thought of as a means to help with either the treatment of addictions or the management of pain. However, as more and more of America's savvy health consumers continue to educate themselves on natural and alternative medicine, more and more of the population is becoming aware that acupuncture can be successfully used as either a main therapy, or an adjunct therapy, for a whole myriad of health issues besides pain management or addiction treatment.

The recognition and acceptance that acupuncture now enjoys in America can all be credited to acupuncture's consistent effectiveness. In particular as it pertains to COPD, there is enough clinical evidence to warrant the use of acupuncture in COPD. Acupuncture has been clinically shown to reduce shortness of breath, improve one's ability to walk, and to improve pulmonary functions testing, to include FEV_1, RV, and TLC. The use of acupuncture in COPD also contributes to a significant overall improvement in quality of life. In some instances, acupuncture may even help to improve one's condition enough such that pharmaceutical medications may either be lessened or possibly eliminated altogether.

Traditional Chinese medicine is based upon the principle that energy (*qi* or *chi*) in the body flows along a series of channels, known as meridians, that run throughout the body. When an individual is healthy, energy is flowing in a balanced manner along these meridians or channels. Consistent also with the concept of energy flow is that when a person is experiencing a diseased state, it is because the energy flow along the meridians has become blocked or disrupted. Acupuncture involves inserting very fine needles into the skin at specific points that lie along these meridians so as to help rebalance the flow of energy (*qi* or *chi*) and promote health.

When performed by a licensed acupuncturist, acupuncture is essentially safe. Some individuals may occasionally feel a slight sensation of pain or bleeding at the needle site, but for the most part, when it is done correctly, acupuncture does not hurt. By using sterile disposable needles, which is for the most part the standard of practice today, infections will be avoided. Appendix 3 contains contact information for the American Association of Oriental Medicine, the Acupuncture and Oriental Medicine Alliance, the National Certification Commission for Acupuncture and Oriental Medicine, and Acufinder. These organizations are all well-respected professional organizations where you can find additional information about acupuncture and traditional Chinese medicine, as well as information on finding a licensed practitioner. Acufinder, in particular, has a very useful website with a lot of general information about acupuncture as well as an extensive database of licensed practitioners. I encourage you to consider using acupuncture as an adjunctive therapy for your COPD. Acupuncture and traditional Chinese medicine are very holistic approaches to healthcare and they will complement any other natural therapeutic protocols you are using. Remember also that most acupuncturists are also trained in Chinese herbal medicine, so you will not only gain the benefit of acupuncture itself but you will avail yourself of all the health benefits that can be gained through the use of Chinese herbs.

Chiropractic

Including chiropractic care in a book such as this is for reasons that are both general and specific. In similar fashion to acupuncture, there has been somewhat of a misperception amongst the American public regarding the role that chiropractic plays in healthcare. Although many people today still only think of chiropractic as being used to address pain, particularly back and neck pain, the fact of the matter is that chiropractic is a complete holistic system of healthcare that is both safe and effective at helping a myriad of health concerns, including COPD.

The crux of chiropractic philosophy lies in understanding how to help correct the health problems that can result from subluxations, or misalignments, of the spine. Essentially, every cell, tissue, and organ in the entire body is ultimately innervated by nerves that pass through the spinal column. When the flow of nerve traffic is interfered with by a misalignment of the spine, many health problems, including back pain, stomach problems, compromised immunity, and respiratory conditions, can occur. Now the fact that you have COPD in and of itself has nothing to do with whether or not your spine is out of adjustment. You got COPD in all likelihood because you smoked, not because your spine is out of adjustment. However, optimizing the alignment of your spine now will allow for the proper and unobstructed flow of nerve transmission to not only your lungs but to every other organ that is involved in trying to restore your body to health. In this fashion, chiropractic is a very holistic means to enhance function, build immunity, and assist the action of the body's innate healing abilities. This is the general reason for including chiropractic care in a book on COPD.

The specific reason for including chiropractic has to do with the mechanics of breathing. Although the sternocleidomastoid has no direct attachments to the spinal column, the diaphragm has attachments to the lumbar vertebrae, and the scalenes have attachments to the cervical vertebrae. Misalignment of the spinal column could affect the optimal functioning of these muscles, especially the diaphragm and the scalenes, since they both have direct attachments to the spinal column. Furthermore, as a consequence of COPD, air often becomes trapped in the lungs and pushes down on the diaphragm. This situation can leave the diaphragm weakened and/or flattened, causing it to work less efficiently such that the neck muscles must then assume an increased share of the work of breathing. This is why it is so important to help in any way possible to maximize the functioning of the breathing muscles.

Chiropractic can clearly help to maintain the spinal column in its proper position, and in so doing it contributes to enabling the muscles of respiration to function optimally. Chiropractic can be especially beneficial in this respect when COPD is severe. Many chiropractors may also be trained in specific techniques that can be used to improve breathing and enhance overall health. Appendix 3 contains information for the National Directory of Chiropractic Foundation, which is a national directory that will enable you to find a chiropractor.

Environmental considerations

Exercising awareness of your environment can play a significant role in reducing or eliminating any potential irritation to your lungs. Individuals with COPD also need to be ever so mindful of their environment so as to minimize factors that contribute to increasing their risk of infections. The following environmental considerations should be taken under advisement and implemented to the extent that it is possible.

- Keep your home or your apartment as clean and dust free as possible. Especially keep your bedroom and your bathroom as clean and dust free as possible. At minimum, a third of your life is spent in your bedroom, so be extra conscious of this room.
- Keep your nebulizer clean and change the tubing often. If you have a suction catheter, keep the container clean and change the tubing often. If you use direct aerosol humidification, keep the machine and the water container clean and definitely change the tubing often.
- Do not use handkerchiefs or cloth towels when taking care of mucus — use tissues or paper towels and dispose of them immediately.
- Reduce clutter as much as possible. This will effectively reduce the surface area for dust and germs.
- Keep trash cans emptied as frequently as possible.

- Use air cleaning machines, both circulating and electrostatic, throughout your home, especially in your bedroom, and change the filters regularly.
- Air conditioning, especially central air conditioning that is filtered, is beneficial for COPD. This is considered essential if you live in a hot and humid climate.
- Use a humidifier as much as possible and be sure to clean the machine frequently to prevent bacterial growth. Humidification is essential for individuals who have thick and copious mucous secretions.
- Use hardwood, ceramic tile, or stone flooring in your home. Carpets contain dirt, dust, chemicals, mold, and many other irritants that are detrimental to your COPD.
- Use wood or plastic blinds as window coverings in your home. Drapes and curtains also contain dirt and dust that are irritating to your lungs.
- The hair and dander of furry or feathered animals are deleterious to your condition.
- Avoid anything that is potentially irritating to the lungs, to include perfumes, colognes, scented laundry products, aerosol products, cleaners, solvents, paint, glue, etc.
- Avoid direct use of gas stoves.
- Do not allow anyone to ever smoke in your home or car.
- Avoid any and all dirty, dusty, or otherwise toxic environments.
- Avoid stressful situations.
- Get plenty of rest and fresh air.

Chapter 8

Final Thoughts

As this book draws to a close, I want to reiterate once more that the foundation of natural therapeutics for COPD is diet and nutrition. Nutrition alone is the cornerstone to everything else that you will ever do therapeutically for COPD. The degree of success you achieve with all other therapeutic methods will always be directly proportional to the effort you make with implementing the dietary and nutritional protocols of chapter 3. If you will change the way you eat by faithfully following all the guidelines of chapter 3, you will without a doubt see a difference in your condition.

The ultimate way to approach things is to first get grounded in modifying your diet. As you begin to become comfortable with new eating patterns and begin to see yourself making progress in improving your condition, you can then begin to make supplements and herbs part of your health building program. Once you have a solid program consisting of diet, supplements, and herbs that has been thoughtfully composed, you will be well on your way to rebuilding your health in a positive direction. Exercise and physical therapeutics will then round out what I consider to be the foundational basics of building health. Diet, supplements, herbs, and exercise are what I consider to be the core ingredients in promoting positive health. By establishing proper eating habits, and assisting your body in its healing processes by supplementing with nutritional supplements and herbs, and by giving your body the exercise it requires, you are giving your body what it needs to function properly as well as removing what are referred to in chapter 7 as obstacles to cure. This is the basis for why natural healthcare is considered to be holistic healthcare. By giving your body these essentials, you not only will be addressing your symptomatic issues with COPD, but you will also be giving your body what it needs in a foundational sense so that it can heal itself. This is one of the central premises of naturopathy — assisting the body in its quest to heal itself.

By creating an optimal internal environment through nutrition, herbs, and exercise, you allow other forms of natural medicine such as homeopathy and acupuncture to be of maximum benefit to you. Natural health, in a lot of ways, is like building a house. You have to start with a solid foundation. The various pieces of natural health like nutrition, herbs, exercise, etc. all build upon each other. You wouldn't try to build the frame of a house before you finished laying a proper foundation. In the same sense, you can't expect to see positive outcome through using homeopathy if you haven't addressed the foundation of your diet.

Be patient and allow your body the time it needs to rebuild itself. Don't expect to see instantaneous results. Quality takes time. I fully understand the frustrations that accompany dealing with COPD everyday. I know you want relief because what you are dealing with everyday makes your life miserable. Not being able to walk more than 5 or 10 feet without having to sit down is no way to live. Not being able to catch your breath, coughing constantly, not being able to work, and always being sick are enough to frustrate any one of us. But there is hope on the horizon. Give yourself an honest 1 to 3 months of following the protocols of this book before you see any significant improvement. Some of you will see improvement after a few weeks to a month, and others will not start seeing any improvement until 3 months or so. I feel confident that if you do what this book says to do, and you work with a healthcare provider who can guide you in the process, you will start to feel better, your symptoms will improve, and you will be well on you way to improved health within a few months.

There are a few specifics that I would like to address before I close. Borage oil is another source of omega–6 gamma–linolenic acid (GLA); however, I have not recommended borage oil because the plant contains pyrrolizidine alkaloids, which are compounds that are potentially toxic to the liver and carcinogenic. Although pyrrolizidine alkaloids are not usually found in the oil, the potential still exists for contamination. As a matter of precaution, and since there are other alternatives that can be used as excellent sources of GLA, I do not recommend using borage oil. For the same reason, I am not recommending the herbs comfrey or coltsfoot. There are plenty of other herbs you can use without taking the unnecessary risks that are associated with these two herbs. I am also not recommending the supplemental omega–3 fish oils EPA and DHA as I feel that it is better in your case to obtain EPA and DHA by consuming the cold–water fishes recommended in chapter 3. Cold–water fish should be a principal component in your diet. Always make sure that you obtain fish from a reliable purveyor that tests its fish to make sure that it does not contain mercury or other undesirable toxins.

Be mindful that as a COPD patient you burn a lot of calories in breathing. The dietary protocols of chapter 3 will enable you to obtain all the calories you need if you maintain proper balance. You may find it more beneficial to eat five or six slightly smaller meals rather than the standard three. Smaller meals with less chewing, eaten more frequently, may make it easier for you to eat enough to still obtain the calories you need and avoid the dyspnea that is often associated with eating big meals.

In closing, I want to wish you well and offer you encouragement as you begin the process to build back your health. This book has been a labor of love as emphysema and COPD are very personal to me. Having experienced it firsthand in my own family has enabled me to empathize with your situation and understand how much you want to get better. Learn as much as you can and get involved as much as possible with others who share your plight. This book is just the beginning for you. As much as I have tried to share with you all that I know about natural health as it pertains to COPD, there is undoubtedly more information that will become available as research continues to reveal new discoveries. Avail yourself of the natural health practitioners that are out there waiting to help you, and never give up hope. My prayers are always with you.

Appendix 1

Standard Conventional Treatment for COPD

The predominant approach of conventional medicine in the treatment of COPD is symptom management. Nursing protocols oftentimes consider holistic methods in addressing the needs of COPD patients, but the overall mainstream approach to treating COPD is through drug management of symptoms. As mentioned in the introduction, some of these drugs may be necessary in the management of COPD in some patients; however, these drugs will not provide any benefit in terms of restorative healing. You may, without any contraindications unless so indicated, implement the nutritional and natural health protocols discussed in this book while remaining on any current medications.

Depending upon the severity of your condition, you will find that if you maintain faithful compliance to the nutritional and natural health protocols discussed in this book, you may very well end up not needing to use as much, if any, pharmaceutical medication. Be mindful though that the cessation of, or the weaning off, of any physician-prescribed medications should always be done under the guidance of your physician or other qualified healthcare provider. Always consult with your physician before you stop taking any prescribed medications. The following are the most commonly prescribed methods used in the treatment of COPD.

Bronchodilators: Bronchodilators are prescribed to provide relaxation of the smooth muscle that surrounds the bronchi and bronchioles. With the relaxation of bronchial smooth muscle, the bronchi and bronchioles can expand and allow for improved airflow. Bronchodilators are classified into three major categories as follows: 1) Short–acting and long–acting beta 2 agonists, 2) Anticholinergic agents, and 3) Methylxanthines.

1) Beta 2 agonists:

Short-acting beta 2 agonists: albuterol, metaproterenol, terbutaline, and pirbuterol. These drugs produce peak bronchodilation at 5–15 minutes and continue to act for 4 to 6 hours.

Long-acting beta 2 agonists: salmeterol, oral sustained-release albuterol. These drugs produce bronchodilation after 15 to 30 minutes and can last up to 12 hours.

2) Anticholinergic agents: ipratropium bromide, tiotropium bromide. By blocking muscarinic receptors, these drugs induce smooth muscle relaxation. Ipratropium acts within 30–60 minutes and can last up to 6 hours. Tiotropium also begins to act within 30–60 minutes but can last up to 24 hours.

3) Methylxanthines: Theophylline. The mechanism of action of theophylline is not fully understood, but it is believed to produce bronchial smooth muscle relaxation by increasing intracellular levels of cAMP through nonspecific phosphodiesterase inhibition. Theophylline is taken orally usually once or twice a day.

Corticosteroids: Corticosteroids are prescribed for their anti–inflammatory properties. Prednisone, the most commonly prescribed corticosteroid, acts as an anti-inflammatory through its inhibition of phospholipase A_2. Prednisone is discussed at length in chapter 3. There are also a variety of inhaled corticosteroids such as budesonide, fluticasone, triamcinolone, and flunisonide.

Expectorants and mucolytics: Expectorants and mucolytics are prescribed for their ability to help thin secretions and move them out of the airway. Guaifenesin is one of the commonly prescribed expectorants; however, guaifenesin is now available over the counter as Mucinex in 600-milligram extended-release tablets. Acetylcysteine is a commonly prescribed mucolytic that is discussed in detail in chapter 4, as acetylcysteine is also considered a nutritional supplement.

Antibiotics: Antibiotics are prescribed for the acute stage of an infection. Because of the recurrent infections of many COPD patients, and the often inappropriate use of antibiotics, many COPD patients become antibiotic resistant, and this can present complications in treatment.

Physical and respiratory therapy: Physical therapy and respiratory therapy involve methods performed by either a physical or respiratory therapist, or a family member who has been trained. These therapies are actually a collection of therapeutic methods whose common goal is to help eliminate mucus from the respiratory tract, enhance respiratory efficiency, and strengthen respiratory muscles. The specific physical therapies for the lungs are deep breathing exercises, coughing, turning, postural drainage, cupping, and vibration. These physical therapies for the lungs are often done in conjunction with other respiratory therapy treatments to rid the airways of secretions. These other treatments include suctioning, nebulizer treatments, aerosol humidification, and the administration of expectorant drugs.

Surgery: In extremely severe cases of COPD, there are three surgical procedures that may be considered.

1. Lung transplant: This is an extremely invasive procedure that is only considered for end-stage COPD patients whose prognosis is worse than the survival statistics for the surgery. Certain specific criteria for FEV_1 and $PaCO_2$ must be met in order to be considered for this surgery.

2. Lung volume reduction surgery: This involves the surgical removal of seriously damaged portions of the lung. Improvement in the elastic recoil of the remaining lung tissue, with concurrent improvement of airflow and exercise capacity, are the goals of this surgery.

3. Bullectomy: A bullectomy is the surgical removal of bullae in the lungs. See chapter 2 for a discussion of bullae. Once the bullae are removed, the healthy air sacs have room to expand, and the muscles used to breathe can function better.

Appendix 2

Smoking Cessation

Most individuals diagnosed with COPD will have, on average, smoked between 150,000 and 400,000 cigarettes and spent around $50,000.00 on cigarettes at the time of their initial diagnosis. Take a moment and ponder those statistics. Great care has been taken throughout this book to elucidate all the damage that is caused by cigarette smoke. Cigarette smoke impairs the sweeping motion of cilia on the respiratory epithelium, which renders the bronchi and larger bronchioles less able to keep themselves clean and free of debris. Cigarette smoke causes hypertrophy and hyperplasia of the mucous-secreting glands that line the respiratory tract. This means that those mucous glands have become enlarged because the cells that comprise them have become enlarged. Cigarette smoke causes the recruitment of neutrophils into the lung. Neutrophils in turn release neutrophil elastase, the enzyme that destroys elastin, which results in destruction of the alveolar wall. Cigarette smoke inhibits the activity of alpha 1 AT, the protein responsible for inhibiting neutrophil elastase. By stimulating irritant receptors in the submucosa of the respiratory tract, cigarette smoke produces smooth muscle constriction that causes an increase in airway resistance. Cigarette smoke causes chronic inflammation in the bronchial wall, and last, but certainly not least, cigarette smoke is irrefutably the main causative agent in lung cancer. And these are just some of the major problems that cigarettes cause in the respiratory system alone. If you were to also consider all the other problems that cigarettes cause in the rest of the body, it should be very apparent by now, especially in light of your diagnosis of COPD, that for your immediate safety and the overall security of your health and life, you must stop smoking now.

You would think that the gravity of a COPD diagnosis alone would be enough to motivate someone to stop smoking. But this is just not the case. Many people face the diagnosis of COPD every day, but not all of them are able to lay down their cigarettes that same day. Some people are able to quit smoking immediately. There is something inside of them that enables them to just do it. Others quit more gradually, and sadly enough, there are those who, despite their illness, take their cigarettes with them to their grave.

I cannot tell you how to stop smoking. I can only tell you that you must stop if you want to have any chance at all in turning your health around. When I finally quit, it was after about a dozen attempts, and it was through using the patch that I was able to finally have success. Whatever method you find that works for you, it will always ultimately come down to your ability to exert your will and simply make the choice not to smoke.

For most smokers, the process of quitting can be a psychological minefield — until you learn *how* to quit. It is only when you try to stop smoking that you become aware of just how many aspects of your life that your smoking habit really dominates. Smoking attaches itself to many subconscious elements of your life. These subconscious attachments reinforce the already strong physiological component of addiction to nicotine. Smoking forms associations to many routine and social aspects of your life such that it becomes problematic in your mind to see yourself participating in certain activities without having a cigarette. Freeing yourself of the psychological bondage brought about by smoking may prove to be very challenging; however, by at least becoming aware of just how many different areas of your life are connected to your smoking habit, you may then begin to envision how your life could be if it was not attached to cigarettes.

There are a variety of tools that can be employed to help you break both the physiological addiction to nicotine as well as the attachments associated with smoking. Some methods may prove more useful than others. Whichever method ends up working for you, it will be because that was the method that was best suited to work in concert with the exercising of your will to stop smoking.

Methods to Assist in Smoking Cessation

Quit Smoking Teleseminars: I highly recommend this smoking cessation program offered by Lela Bryan. Since 1978, Lela has helped thousands of individuals to learn how to permanently kick the habit. Of the people who complete her course, 90 percent of them quit smoking. The long-term success rate is around 70 percent. Information on her well-established and critically acclaimed smoking cessation program can be obtained on the Internet at **www.quitsmokingteleseminars. com**, or by calling toll free 1-800-800-4472.

Acupuncture: The effectiveness of acupuncture in treating addictions is very well recognized. Acupuncture has well-established success rates with cigarette addiction. Appendix 3 contains information to find a qualified acupuncturist.

Hypnosis: This is a technique that has been used successfully by many smokers to kick the habit. Be sure to find a hypnotherapist who has experience in smoking cessation. Appendix 3 contains information to find a qualified hypnotherapist.

Homeopathy: There is no specific homeopathic remedy for smoking cessation, but a skilled homeopathic practitioner can be very helpful in selecting a remedy that will be useful in helping you achieve your overall comprehensive healing goals, of which smoking cessation is a part. Refer to the section on homeopathy in chapter 7 for a review of the basic principles upon which homeopathic therapeutics are based. Appendix 3 contains information to find a qualified homeopathic practitioner.

Herbal medicine: Herbs that have been found to be useful in smoking cessation are lobelia, American angelica, black cohosh, blue cohosh, blue vervain, catnip, echinacea, ginseng, hyssop, motherwort, peppermint, skullcap, slippery elm, and valerian. These herbs exert varying effects that will ease the process of smoking cessation. A combination formula made by combining the liquid extracts of oat seed (50%), licorice root

(25%), and lobelia (25%) can be useful in overcoming tobacco addiction. Appendix 3 contains information to find a qualified herbalist.

Nicotine patches/nicotine gum: With the nonprescription availability of nicotine patches and gum, these two aids for smoking cessation have risen in popularity. This is the method that I personally used with success, but bear in mind that this method, although it will help greatly to alleviate the physical cravings for nicotine, still requires a great amount of effort and will power.

Nicotine vaccine: Although it is not yet available for the public, Swiss researchers reported in May of 2005 that an experimental vaccine against nicotine helped smokers to stop smoking. The experimental testing of heavy smokers indicated that 40 percent of them were able to quit for six months after receiving the vaccine. Much more testing is required, but Zurich-based Cytos Biotechnology hopes to have the vaccine on the market by 2010.

Hospital-based programs: Most hospitals regularly sponsor smoking cessation programs. Contact your local hospital for further information.

Appendix 3

Additional Resources

The organizations listed in this appendix are offered as a convenience to assist you with obtaining further information, products, and practitioner referrals. The organizations listed are generally well reputed, but always use your own discretion to determine the suitability of any particular organization, company, or practitioner to serve your needs.

Nutrition Professionals

American Association of Nutritional Consultants

AANC
401 Kings Highway
Winona Lake, IN 46590
888-828-2262
www.aanc.net

National Association of Nutrition Professionals

NANP
P.O. Box 971
Veradale, WA 99037
800-342-8037
www.nanp.org

Price–Pottenger Nutrition Foundation

P.O. Box 2614
La Mesa, CA 91943
619-462-7600
www.price–pottenger.org

Herbalists and Botanical Medicine Information

American Herbalists Guild

AHG
141 Nob Hill Road
Cheshire, CT 06410
203-272-6731
www.americanherbalistsguild.com

American Botanical Council

P.O. Box 144345
Austin, TX 78714-4345
512-926-4900
www.herbalgram.org

Physicians (M.D. and D.O.)

American Holistic Medical Association

AHMA
12101 Menaul Blvd. NE
Suite C
Albuquerque, NM 87112
505-292-7788
www.holisticmedicine.org

American College for Advancement in Medicine

ACAM
23121 Verdugo Drive, Suite 204
Laguna Hills, CA 92653
888-439-6891
www.acam.org

Naturopaths and Holistic Health Practitioners

American Naturopathic Medical Association

ANMA
P.O. Box 96273
Las Vegas, NV 89193
702-897-7053
www.anma.com

American Association of Drugless Practitioners
American Alternative Medical Association

AADP & AAMA
2200 Market Street
Suite 329
Galveston, TX 77550
409-621-2600
www.aadp.net
www.joinaama.com

American Holistic Health Association

AHHA
P.O. Box 17400
Anaheim, CA 92817
714-779-6152
www.ahha.org

National Association of Certified Natural Health Professionals

CNHP
712 East Winona Avenue
Warsaw, IN 46580
800-321-1005
www.cnhp.org

Homeopathic Practitioners

National Center for Homeopathy
801 N. Fairfax Street, Suite 306
Alexandria, VA 22314
703-548-7790
877-624-0613
www.homeopathic.org

North American Society of Homeopaths
NASH
P.O. Box 450039
Sunrise, FL 33345
206-720-7000
www.homeopathy.org

Acupuncture and Oriental Medicine

American Association of Oriental Medicine
AAOM
P.O. Box 162340
Sacramento, CA 95816
916-443-4770
www.aaom.org

Acufinder.com
825 College Blvd
Suite 102–211
Oceanside, CA 92057
760-630-3600
www.acufinder.com

National Certification Commission for
Acupuncture & Oriental Medicine

NCCAOM
11 Canal Center Plaza
Suite 300
Alexandria, VA 22314
703-548-9004
www.nccaom.org

Acupuncture & Oriental Medicine Alliance

AOMA
6405 43rd Avenue Ct NW
Suite A
Gig Harbor, WA 98335
253-851-6896
www.acuall.org

Chiropractors

National Directory of Chiropractic Foundation

406 E 300 South
Box 305
Salt Lake City, UT 84111
800-888-7914
www.chirodirectory.com

Hypnotherapists

National Guild of Hypnotists

NGH
P.O. Box 308
Merrimack, NH 03054
603-429-9438
www.ngh.net

Products and Services

Source for nebulizer equipment

Allergy Be Gone
34 34th Street, Unit 3
Brooklyn, NY 11232
866-234-6630
www.allergybegone.com
Alan Barsano

Source for nebulizer glutathione

Medaus Pharmacy & Compounding Center
2637 Valleydale Road
Suite 200
Birmingham, AL 35244
800-526-9183
www.medaus.com
Larry Stephens or Steven Russell

Source for colloidal silver

Purest Colloids, Inc.
213 Irick Road
Westhampton, NJ 08060
609-267-6284
www.purestcolloids.com
Frank Key

Source for bulk herbs

Mountain Rose Herbs
P.O. Box 50220
Eugene, OR 97405
800-879-3337
www.mountainroseherbs.com

Sources for herbal liquid extracts
Nature's Answer
75 Commerce Drive
Hauppauge, NY 11788
800-439-2324
www.naturesanswer.com

Eclectic Institute, Inc.
36350 SE Industrial Way
Sandy, OR 97055
800-332-4372
www.eclecticherb.com
www.eclecticwater.com

Wise Woman Herbals, Inc.
P.O. Box 279
Creswell, OR 97426
541-895-5172
www.wisewomanherbals.com

Other Practitioners and Information

International Association of Yoga Therapists   (Practitioners)
IAYT
P.O. Box 2513
Prescott, AZ 86302
928-541-0004
www.iayt.org

American Massage Therapy Association   (Practitioners)
500 Davis St., Suite 900
Evanston, IL 60201
888-843-2682
www.amtamassage.org

International Society for Orthomolecular
Medicine   (Information)
ISOM
16 Florence Avenue
Toronto, Ontario
Canada M2N 1E9
416-733-2117
www.orthomed.org

American Physical Therapy Association   (Practitioners)
APTA
1111 N. Fairfax Street
Alexandria, VA 22314
800-999-2782
703-684-2782
www.apta.org

Selected Bibliography

Alberts, Bruce, et al. *Molecular Biology of the Cell.* 4th ed. New York: Garland Science, 2002.

Anderson, Kenneth N., Lois E. Anderson, and Walter D. Glanze, eds. *Mosby's Medical, Nursing, & Allied Health Dictionary.* 4th ed. St. Louis, MO: Mosby, 1994.

Balch, Phyllis, A., and James F. Balch. *Prescription for Nutritional Healing.* 3rd ed. New York: Avery, 2000.

Bellavite, Paolo, and Andrea Signorini. *The Emerging Science of Homeopathy — Complexity, Biodynamics, and Nanopharmacology.* Berkeley, CA: North Atlantic Books, 2002.

Braunwald, Eugene, et al. *Harrison's Principles of Internal Medicine.* 15th ed. New York: McGraw-Hill, 2001.

Champe, Pamela C., Richard A. Harvey, and Denise R. Ferrier. *Lippincott's Illustrated Reviews: Biochemistry.* 3rd ed. Philadelphia: Lippincott, Williams, & Wilkins, 2005.

Chandra, V., Jayasankar Jasti, Punit Kaur, Ch. Betzel, A. Srinivasan, and T.P. Singh. "First Structural Evidence of a Specific Inhibitor of Phospholipase A_2 by α–tocopherol (vitamin E) and Its Implications in Inflammation: Crystal Structure of the Complex Formed Between Phospholipase A_2 and α–tocopherol at 1.8 Å Resolution." *Journal of Molecular Biology.* 320 (2002): 215–222.

Cooper, Geoffrey M. *The Cell: A Molecular Approach.* Sunderland, England: Sinauer Associates, 1997.

Cotran, Ramzi S., Vinay Kumar, and Tucker Collins. *Robbins Pathologic Basis of Disease.* 6th ed. Philadelphia: W.B. Saunders, 1999.

Grippi, Michael A. *Pulmonary Pathophysiology.* Philadelphia: Lippincott, Williams, & Wilkins, 1995.

Gruenwald, Joerg, Thomas Brendler, and Christof Jaenicke, eds. *PDR for Herbal Medicines.* 2nd ed. Montvale, NJ: Thomson Healthcare, 2000.

Guyton, Arthur C., and John E. Hall. *Textbook of Medical Physiology.* 10th ed. Philadelphia: W.B. Saunders, 2000.

Hendler, Sheldon S., and David Rorvik, eds. *PDR for Nutritional Supplements.* Montvale, NJ: Thomson Healthcare, 2001.

Lust, John. *The Herb Book.* New York: Bantam Books, 1974.

Lust, John, and Michael Tierra. *The Natural Remedy Bible.* New York: Pocket Books, 1990.

Murray, Michael, and Joseph Pizzorno. *Encyclopedia of Natural Medicine.* 2nd ed. Rocklin, CA: Prima Health, 1998.

Netter, Frank H. *Atlas of Human Anatomy.* 2nd ed. East Hanover, NJ: Novartis, 1997.

Pedersen, Mark. *Nutritional Herbology.* Warsaw, IN: Wendell W. Whitman Company, 2002.

Pentland, Alice P., Aubrey R. Morrison, Susan C. Jacobs, Luciann Lisi Hruza, Jason S. Hebert, and Lester Packer. "Tocopherol Analogs Suppress Arachidonic Acid Metabolism via Phospholipase Inhibition." *Journal of Biological Chemistry.* 267 (1992): 15578–15584.

Price, Silvia Anderson, and Lorraine McCarty Wilson. *Pathophysiology — Clinical Concepts of Disease Process.* 4th ed. St. Louis, MO: Mosby Year Book, 1992.

Smith, Ed. *Therapeutic Herb Manual.* Williams, OR: Ed Smith, 1999.

Stryer, Lubert. *Biochemistry.* 4th ed. New York: W.H. Freeman & Company, 1995.

Taddei-Ferretti, C., and P. Marotta, eds. *High Dilution Effects on Cells and Integrated Systems.* London: World Scientific, 1998.

Tierra, Michael. *Planetary Herbology.* Twin Lakes, WI: Lotus Press, 1992.

Traves, Suzanne L., and Louise E. Donnelly. "Chemokines and Their Receptors as Targets for the Treatment of COPD." *Current Respiratory Medicine Reviews.* 1 (2005): 15–32.

Tortora, Gerard J., and Sandra Reynolds Grabowski. *Principles of Anatomy and Physiology.* 7th ed. New York: HarperCollins, 1993.

Trivieri Jr., Larry, and John W. Anderson, eds. *Alternative Medicine — The Definitive Guide.* Berkeley, CA: Celestial Arts, 2002.

Uthe, J., and W. Magee. "Phospholipase A2: Action as Affected by Deoxycholate and Divalent Cations." *Canadian Journal of Biochemistry.* 49 (1971): 776–784.

West, John B. *Pulmonary Pathophysiology: The Essentials.* 6th ed. Philadelphia: Lippincott, Williams, & Wilkins, 2003.

Zuidema, George D., ed. *The Johns Hopkins Atlas of Human Functional Anatomy.* 4th ed. Baltimore, MD: Johns Hopkins University Press, 1997.

Glossary

Acute — Acute is used to describe an illness that begins abruptly with marked intensity, but then subsides after a relatively short period of time. Compare acute with chronic.

Antioxidant — An antioxidant is a substance that works to prevent damage to the body's cells from free radicals. The normal cellular processes of oxidation in our bodies produce highly reactive free radicals. Free radicals are also contained in cigarette smoke. COPD patients have significant amounts of oxidative damage in their lungs due to free radicals. Free radicals readily react with and damage other molecules and cells. Antioxidants are capable of "mopping up" free radicals before they damage other essential molecules or cells.

Anti–protease — An anti–protease is a protein that has the capability of inhibiting the activity of a protease. Alpha 1 antitrypsin is an anti–protease that inhibits the activity of the protease neutrophil elastase.

Antitussive — An antitussive is a substance, oftentimes an herb, that helps to relieve coughing.

Atrophy — Atrophy is when there is wasting, or diminution of size or physiologic activity, of a part of the body because of disease or other influences.

Atypical — Atypical refers to when a situation or condition is different from what would be considered the usual, or typical type.

Carminative — A carminative is a substance, oftentimes an herb, that helps to relieve gas in the stomach and the bowels.

Catalyst — A catalyst is a substance, usually an enzyme when referring to a biological system, that influences the rate of a chemical reaction without becoming consumed or permanently altered in the process.

Cation — A cation is a positively charged ion. It is an atom that has lost electrons such that it becomes a positively charged ion.

Chemotactic — Chemotactic refers to the tendency of cells to migrate either toward or away from a chemical stimulus.

Chemotaxis — Chemotaxis refers to a response that involves movement either toward or away from a chemical stimulus.

Chemotactic, chemotaxis, and chemotactic factors — These words describe phenomena involving chemical attractions. Consider this further explanation by way of an example: Alveolar macrophages (immune cells in the alveoli) release neutrophil chemotactic (attraction) factors, which are simply molecules that cause the increased recruitment of neutrophils into the lung. In other words, **chemotactic (attraction) factors** are molecules released from macrophages that attract **(chemotaxis)** neutrophils to come into the lungs. If a substance such as nicotine is **chemotactic (causes attraction)** for neutrophils, this means that the very presence of nicotine will cause increased recruitment of neutrophils into the lungs.

Chronic — Chronic refers to a disease or disorder that develops slowly and persists over a long period of time.

Cilia (Ciliated) — Cilia are small hairlike structures on the outer surfaces of some cells. Some of the respiratory epithelium contains cilia, which aid in the process of removing mucus and debris from the respiratory tract.

Connective tissue — Connective tissue is one of the fundamental tissue types found in the human body. There are several types of connective tissue, one of which is loose connective tissue, which functions to hold organs and epithelia in place. Loose connective tissue contains a variety of fibers to include collagen and elastin.

Contraindication — A contraindication is any factor that would prohibit the use of a drug, supplement, herb, or other therapeutic method.

Cytokines — Cytokines are small protein molecules that act as messengers between cells of the immune system, and between immune system cells and other cell types.

Cytoplasm — The cytoplasm is essentially all the internal contents contained within a cell except for the nucleus. It is a jelly–like material that consists mainly of water. The cytoplasm contains all of the cell's organelles along with salts, organic molecules, and many enzymes.

Diaphoretic — A diaphoretic is a substance, oftentimes an herb, that promotes perspiration.

Distal — Distal refers to being away from, or being farthest from a point of origin.

Dysplasia — Dysplasia refers to any abnormal development or cellular changes, such as alterations in size, shape, or organization of cells that occur within tissues or organs.

Edema — Edema refers to the abnormal accumulation of fluid in the interstitial spaces of tissues. Interstitial spaces are the spaces between tissues.

Elastase, neutrophil lysosomal — Elastase is an enzyme from the class of proteases that break down proteins. Specifically as it pertains to this book, neutrophil elastase is a protease that breaks down the protein elastin in the interalveolar septum (alveolar wall).

Elastin (elastic fibers) — Elastin is a protein that is the principal constituent of elastic tissue fibers. These are the elastic fibers that are found in the interalveolar septum (alveolar wall) that are destroyed by the enzyme neutrophil elastase.

Enzyme — An enzyme is a protein that is produced by living cells that acts as a catalyst for the chemical reactions that occur within the organism. Most enzymes catalyze reactions that occur within the cell.

Epithelium (epithelial cells) — Epithelium is one of the four fundamental tissues of the human body. Epithelial tissue is composed of a layer of cells that can be found covering body surfaces; lining hollow organs, body cavities, and ducts; and forming glands. Epithelium includes the cells that line the inside of the respiratory tract.

Expectorant — An expectorant is a substance, oftentimes an herb, that helps facilitate the removal of mucus and phlegm from the bronchial passageways.

Fibrosis — Fibrosis refers to the proliferation of fibrous connective tissue. The process of fibrosis is a normal process in the formation of scar tissue that replaces normal tissue that is lost through injury or infection; however, it can become abnormal when the fibrous connective tissue spreads over or replaces normal smooth muscle or other normal organ tissue.

Flavonoids — Flavonoids are low-molecular-weight phytochemicals found in vascular plants. They exert a wide range of biological effects to include antioxidant and anti–inflammatory effects.

Gluten — Gluten is a protein found in wheat. It is a sticky, elastic substance that is formed when gliadin and glutenin, two insoluble proteins also found in wheat, are combined when wheat is moistened and kneaded.

Goblet cells — A goblet cell is one of the specialized cells that secrete mucus and form glands of the epithelium of the respiratory tract, stomach, and intestines.

Hemoglobin — Hemoglobin is a complex iron-containing protein molecule contained within red blood cells that enables them to bind and carry oxygen.

Histamine — Histamine is a protein that acts as a chemical transmitter that is involved in local immune responses, regulation of stomach acid production, and in allergic reactions as a mediator of hypersensitivity. It causes an inflammatory response as well as the contraction of smooth muscle, which induces bronchoconstriction.

Holistic — *Holistic* can have a variety of connotations, but as it is implied in this book, it refers to having an approach to health and living that considers the entirety of an individual's well–being. This includes addressing the physical, mental, and emotional aspects of an individual as well as promoting the nutritional and lifestyle modifications that will lead to a healthy existence.

Inhibitor — An inhibitor is a supplement, herb, drug, or other agent that prevents or restricts a certain action. Many of the inhibitors discussed in this book are substances that prevent or restrict the activity of certain enzymes.

Labyrinth — A labyrinth is a structure that contains an intricate and complicated network of winding passages that is hard to follow without losing one's way.

Laryngectomee — A laryngectomee is a person who has surgically lost his or her larynx, usually due to cancer.

Leukocyte — Leukocyte is the generic overall name given for white blood cells. Leukocytes are subdivided into lymphocytes, monocytes, neutrophils, basophils, and eosinophils.

Lipid peroxidation — Lipid peroxidation is defined as the oxidative deterioration of lipids as a result of oxidative stress. Lipid peroxidation is a free radical–related process that causes cellular damage.

Lymphocyte — A lymphocyte is a type of white blood cell (leukocyte) that develops in the bone marrow and plays an integral part in the body's defenses. Lymphocytes occur as B cells, which are involved in antigen-antibody immune responses (humoral immunity), and T cells, which are involved in cell-mediated immunity.

Metaplasia — Metaplasia is the conversion of normal tissue cells into an abnormal form in response to chronic stress or injury. See dysplasia.

Mucolytic — A mucolytic is a substance that dissolves or destroys mucus.

Mucous membrane — Mucous membranes are thin layers of tissue that line or cover the cavities or canals of the body that are open to the outside. Mucous membranes line the respiratory passages, the digestive tract, and the urogenital tract. Mucous membranes consist of a surface layer of epithelium that covers a deeper layer of connective tissue.

Naturopath (N.D.) — A naturopath is an individual who has completed a curriculum of study and has been awarded the doctor of naturopathy (N.D.) degree. Traditional naturopaths are primarily teachers who educate clients on approaches to healthful living and building health through noninvasive natural means. Traditional naturopaths may help individuals overcome their health issues through dietary/nutritional modification, nutritional supplements, herbs and botanicals, bodywork, hydrotherapy, exercise or body movement, and prayer or meditation. Naturopathy itself is a philosophy of life and an approach to living. It involves living a lifestyle as close to nature as possible, which includes consuming food derived from natural sources, drinking pure water, breathing fresh air, enjoying the warmth of sunshine, exercising the body regularly in natural ways, and obtaining adequate rest. True naturopathy never involves the use of drugs, surgery, or any invasive procedures.

Necrosis — Necrosis refers to the localized tissue death that occurs in groups of cells in response to injury or disease.

Nucleus — The nucleus is the command center of the cell. It is the organelle that contains the genetic material that is necessary to maintain the functions of the cell.

Pathogenesis — Pathogenesis refers to the cause or causes of an illness.

Pathogenic — If something is said to be pathogenic, it is because it is capable of causing or producing a disease or illness.

pH — a measure of the relative acidity or alkalinity of a solution. pH is measured on a scale of 0–14 with 7 being neutral, less than 7 being acidic, and greater than 7 being alkaline or basic.

Phagocytosis — Phagocytosis is the process by which certain cells engulf and destroy microorganisms and cellular debris.

Polymorphonuclear — Having a multi–lobed nucleus such as a neutrophil. A neutrophil is a polymorphonuclear leukocyte.

Prophylactically — Prophylactically is the word used to describe when something is done as a preventative measure.

Protease — A protease is an enzyme that breaks down proteins. See elastase.

Proteolysis — Proteolysis is the enzymatic process of breaking down a protein.

Reducing agent — A reducing agent is a substance that donates electrons to another substance in a chemical reaction.

Smooth muscle — Smooth muscle is a type of muscle tissue that is not under voluntary control. It lacks cross striations on its fibers and is found principally with the internal organs. Smooth muscle surrounds the bronchi and bronchioles of the respiratory tract.

Subepithelial — Subepithelial refers to the area beneath the epithelium.

Submucosal — Submucosal refers to the layer of loose connective tissue beneath a mucous membrane.

Synapse — The synapse is the area between two nerve cells, or between a nerve cell and an organ or muscle, across which nerve impulses are transmitted through the action of a neurotransmitter.

Synergy (Synergistic) — Synergy is the process whereby two or more substances work together simultaneously to enhance the function and effect of one another. When nutritional protocols and herbs, for example, are used to enhance health, they have a synergistic effect in the sense that they work together to not only address symptoms per se, but to aid in improving the overall health status of the body.

Therapeutic — Therapeutic refers to something that is beneficial as a healing agent, or that has healing properties.

Thoracic cavity — The thoracic cavity consists of the structures enclosed by the ribs (heart, lungs, muscles, etc.), the thoracic portion of the vertebral column, the sternum, and the diaphragm.

Tonic — A tonic is a substance, oftentimes an herb, that helps to restore normal tone and function to the tissues of the body.

Index

A

C

O

P

Vitamins
    B complex 121, 124
    C 108, 111-112, 114-116, 124
    E – see (d – α – tocopherol)
    K 108
    Multi 121, 124

W

Walking 7, 150
Water 6, 32-33, 35, 43, 80-81, 84, 86, 93-97, 112, 116-117, 120, 132-147, 158, 167, 191, 194
Wheat 81, 84, 86, 192
Wheezing 136, 155
White blood cells 54, 62-63, 78, 193
    Eosinophil(s) 62, 193
    Leukocytes(s) 63, 78-79, 85, 193
        Polymorphonuclear 105, 133
    Lymphocyte(s) 62-63, 193-194
    Neutrophil(s) 53-58, 62, 79, 104, 135, 173, 189-191, 193, 195
White flour 81, 85-86
Wild cherry 116, 143-144, 147

Y

Yarrow 144, 146-147
Yerba santa 116, 143
Yoga 7, 150, 152-153, 183

Z

Zinc 109-110, 124